CONTENTS

KV-142-138

Section 1. General
1. Acute cutaneous infections — 02
2. Specific infections — 05
3. Burns — 09
4. Postoperative complications — 13
5. Neck — 19
6. Breast — 24

Section 2. Skin, its Adnexae and Subcutaneous Tissues
7. Benign conditions — 38
8. Benign and malignant tumours — 43

Section 3. Oromaxillofacial
9. Facial fractures — 60
10. Oral cavity — 64
11. Salivary glands — 77
12. Pharynx — 82

Section 4. Thorax
13. Lungs and chest wall — 86
14. Heart and great vessels — 92
15. Mediastinum — 100
16. Oesophagus — 103
17. Diaphragmatic hernias — 110

Section 5. Abdomen
18. The acute abdomen — 116
19. Stomach and duodenum — 121
20. Liver — 132
21. Gallbladder and bile ducts — 146
22. Pancreas — 159
23. Spleen — 173
24. Specific and special forms of obstruction — 178
25. Small bowel and appendix — 187
26. Colon — 197
27. Anal canal and rectum — 209

28. Hernia   218
29. Surgical gynaecology   227

Section 6. Vascular
30. Occlusive arterial disease   232
31. Aneurysmal arterial disease   247
32. Veins and lymphatics   253

Section 7. Endocrinology
33. Thyroid and parathyroid   266
34. Adrenal   275

Section 8. Urology
35. Kidney and ureter   282
36. Bladder and prostate   295
37. Urethra and penis   299
38. Testis   303

Section 9. Neurology
39. Brain and meninges   310
40. Head injuries   319
41. Spinal cord   325
42. Peripheral nerve injuries   331

Index   339

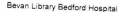

Color Atlas of

SURGICAL DIAGNOSIS

Mr J. Donald Greig
MB ChB MD FRCS (Ed. & Glasg.) FRCS (Gen.)
Consultant Surgeon
St John's Hospital, Livingston
and
Honorary Senior Lecturer
University of Edinburgh

Mr O. James Garden
BSc MB ChB MD FRCS (Ed. & Glasg.)
Senior Lecturer
University of Edinburgh
and
Honorary Consultant Surgeon
Royal Infirmary, Edinburgh

M Mosby-Wolfe

London Baltimore Barcelona Bogotá Boston Buenos Aires Caracas Carlsbad, CA Chicago Madrid Mexico City Milan Naples, FL New York
Philadelphia St. Louis Seoul Singapore Sydney Taipei Tokyo Toronto Wiesbaden

Publisher:	Geoff Greenwood
Development Editor:	Lucy Hamilton
Project Managers:	Linda Kull
	Emma Dorey
Editorial Assistant:	Sarah Edwards
Production:	Siobhan Egan
Index:	Michael Robertson
Layout:	Martyn Oliver

Preface

It has become apparent to us, over recent years, that fewer opportunities exist for the medical undergraduate and postgraduate student to observe the full range of 'general' surgery. With increasing surgical specialisation and changes in working practice, the traditional attachment to one surgical firm may only provide exposure to a limited surgical field. Furthermore, the increasing trend towards day case surgery and outpatient treatment may leave the student with a rather unbalanced view of common surgical pathology. The student may therefore feel unprepared to face the surgical examiner and, more importantly, may be poorly equipped to go into general practice and deal with these clinical problems.

This textbook has been produced in an attempt to provide the student and the medical graduate with a general overview of surgical practice. The emphasis is on the demonstration of clinical signs but, where appropriate, we have endeavoured to guide the reader through the relevant diagnostic and therapeutic pathway. We have resisted the temptation to use this project as a means of dusting down our respective slide collections and focusing on surgical rarities. Similarly, we have attempted to strike a balance between the use of clinical photographs and radiographs, but we recognise that in some areas of the book, such as in the vascular and thoracic sections, the use of radiographs provides a more rounded view of surgical practice. The text is not comprehensive but rather focuses on key areas of surgical relevance. Nonetheless, we hope that the detailed descriptions that accompany many of the illustrations will give the reader a firm understanding of the management of common surgical conditions. Whereas the undergraduate will undoubtedly find this to be of considerable help in negotiating the examination hurdle, we have also intended that the atlas will be of use to the postgraduate and general practitioner in keeping abreast of current surgical practice.

J. Donald Greig
O. James Garden

ACKNOWLEDGMENTS

This book would not have been possible without the help of a number of individuals and the authors are indebted to the following colleagues who have provided us with slides to fill in the gaps in some of the clinical sections: Dr. J. Bell (Consultant Neuropathologist, Edinburgh); Mr. Michael Brockbank (Consultant ENT Surgeon, Salisbury); Professor David Carter (Regius Professor of Surgery, Edinburgh); Professor Geoffrey Chisholm, (Consultant Urologist, Edinburgh); Mr. Michael Dixon (Consultant Breast Surgeon, Edinburgh); Dr. Hugh Gilmour (Consultant Pathologist, Edinburgh); Dr. Michael Hendry (Consultant Paediatric Radiologist, Edinburgh); Mr. David Lee (Consultant Surgeon, Edinburgh); Dr. Keith Little (Consultant in Accident and Emergency Medicine, Edinburgh); Mr. Iain Macintyre (Consultant General Surgeon, Edinburgh); Dr. Margaret Macintyre (Consultant Pathologist, Edinburgh); Mr. William McKerrow (Consultant ENT Surgeon, Inverness); Mr. Stephen Nixon (Consultant General Surgeon, Edinburgh); Mr. John O'Neill (Consultant Surgeon, Melrose); Dr. Doris Redhead (Consultant Radiologist, Edinburgh); W Hamish Thomson and Oxford University Press (for Fig. 27.3, left); Professor Vaughn Ruckley (Consultant Vascular Surgeon, Edinburgh); Mr. William Walker (Consultant Cardiothoracic Surgeon, Edinburgh); Mr. James Watson (Consultant Plastic Surgeon, Livingston); and Mr. Graham Wilson (Consultant General Surgeon, Edinburgh).

We are also particularly grateful to the following colleagues who gave up a little more of their time in revising chapters or sections and updating clinical material that we felt needed specialist input to ensure that our own thoughts were in line with optimal surgical practice: Mr. Andrew Bradbury (Senior Registrar in Vascular Surgery, Edinburgh: Section 6); Mr. Michael Dixon (Consultant Breast Surgeon, Edinburgh: Chapter 6); Mr. Douglas Gentleman (Consultant Neurosurgeon, Dundee: Section 9); Mr. Graham Haddock (Senior Registrar in Paediatric Surgery, Glasgow: Paediatric and Neonatal material); Mr. Roy Mitchell (Consultant Oromaxillofacial Surgeon, Edinburgh: Section 3; and Mr. Richard Stevenson (Senior Registrar in Urology, Edinburgh: Section 8).

We are indebted to Eileen Currie, Anne McKellar, Carole Tomlinson, Susan Rowley and Monica McGill for their help in preparing manuscripts, and to Ian Lennox for his assistance in providing us with some of the illustrations.

Finally, we are grateful to Geoff Greenwood and Lucy Hamilton of Mosby-Wolfe who have guided, encouraged and coerced us into producing this textbook. We trust that the final product will be more than a useful addition to their already established series of clinical atlases.

Section 1

General

1.

ACUTE CUTANEOUS INFECTIONS

The organisms responsible for most skin infections are the Gram positive *Staphylococcus* (*S.*) and *Streptococcus species*. As a general principle, antibiotics are invaluable for treating infections which are spreading through tissues, but drainage with and without tissue debridement is required when abscess formation has occurred. Prior to commencement of antimicrobial therapy, pus obtained by aspiration, surgical wound swab or blood should be cultured. If the infection is life-threatening then 'best guess' antimicrobial treatment should be commenced, and subsequently altered, if required, when identification and antibiotic sensitivities of the organism become available.

Diagnosis

The **cardinal signs** are **pyrexia**, localised **pain**, **erythema**, **oedema** and, if an abscess has developed, **fluctuation** and **induration** may also be present. The development of a spreading infection, tissue crepitus, systemic toxicity or cardiovascular instability signal severe infection which must be recognised and dealt with aggressively.

S. aureus is the most common isolate from subcutaneous abscesses, gaining access by local tissue trauma or skin penetration, and is responsible for furuncles, carbuncles, web space infections and suppurative tenosynovitis. Other infective pathogens such as viruses, yeasts, fungi and protozoa should be considered in the differential diagnosis. If pus is present, drainage or repeated aspiration is mandatory. Frequent skin infections suggest possible co-existent disease, such as diabetes mellitus, vascular impairment or renal insufficiency.

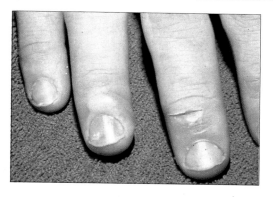

1.1 Paronychia. An infection of the nail bed caused by *S. aureus*. This required surgical incision under digital block anaesthesia to release the pus.

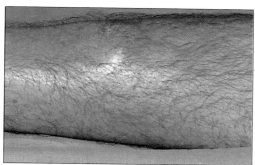

1.2 Folliculitis. An early *S. aureus* infection which was initially treated by oral flucloxacillin for 48 hours. The obvious development of an abscess with cellulitis necessitated subsequent surgical drainage.

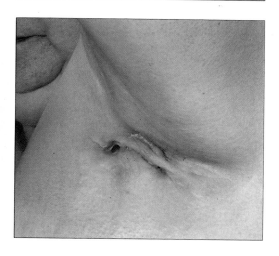

1.3 Hydradenitis suppurativa. Recurrent *S. aureus* infection of axillary apocrine glands is usually responsible for this condition. It may also frequently affect the groin area. Although multiple drainage procedures can be undertaken, frequency of infection is an indication for definitive excision of apocrine-bearing skin in the affected areas, with primary closure or skin grafting if necessary.

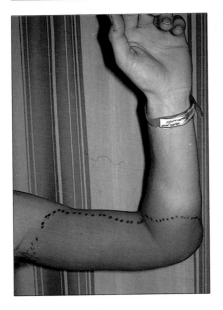

1.4 Erysipelas. This is a spreading subcutaneous skin infection caused by *beta-haemolytic Streptococci*. There is an associated lymphangitis and septicaemia in the absence of pus. Following treatment with high-dose parenteral penicillin, the cellulitis resolved after seven days.

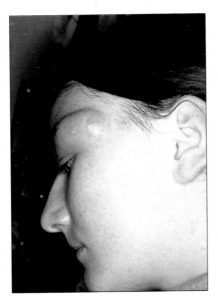

1.5 Streptococcal periorbital cellulitis. The cellulitis flared up within four hours of the patient's attempt to expurgate a facial spot. Failure to recognise and treat this infection urgently and aggressively may result in cavernous sinus thrombosis.

2.

SPECIFIC INFECTIONS

TETANUS

Tetanus is caused by *Clostridium tetani* and follows the implantation of spores into a deep, devitalised wound. The exotoxin produced by the organism acts upon the motor cells of the central nervous system. The incubation time ranges from 24 hours to 24 days. Muscle spasm develops at the site of innoculation and then involves the facial muscles. It is the trismus of the facial spasm which produces 'lock-jaw'. The period of spasm is followed by convulsion.

Prophylaxis against this condition is achieved by active immunisation with tetanus toxoid (two injections at an interval of 6 weeks) and the administration of a booster dose at intervals of not less than 5 years.

Treatment involves the controlling of convulsions, eradication of local infection, and maintenance of the electrolyte balance.

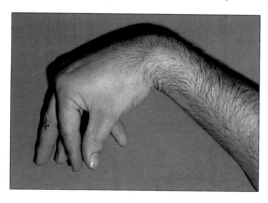

2.1 Tetanic spasm of the right hand. Despite attempts to control convulsions, excision of the wound and administration of human gamma globulin, this patient did not respond to treatment.

ACTINOMYCOSIS

This infection is produced by the *Actinomyces* fungus and may give rise to intra-oral sepsis following dental extraction or tonsillitis, with spread to the cervical region. It has been associated with infection of the ileocaecal region following perforated appendicitis and may give rise to severe pulmonary infection. Treatment consists of prolonged treatment with pencillin.

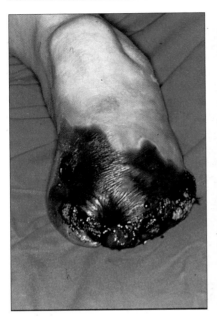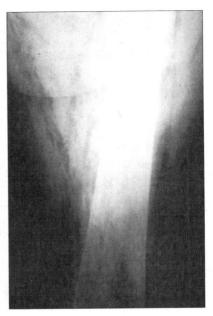

2.2 Gas gangrene. This below-the-knee amputation stump shows gross evidence of gas gangrene (*left*). Alternatively, radiography may also demonstrate gas in the soft tissues from the anaerobic infection (*right*). Treatment with penicillin is accompanied by radical excision of all involved tissue, even if this necessitates amputation.

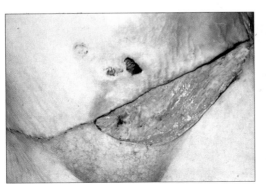

2.3 Necrotising fasciitis. Diffuse discoloration of skin overlying the necrotic fascia and fat of the perineum, caused principally by a *beta-haemolytic Streptococcus*. In this patient there has been inadequate initial debridement of the infected wound, with superior extension of the aggressive infection.

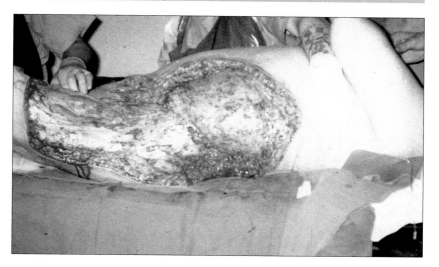

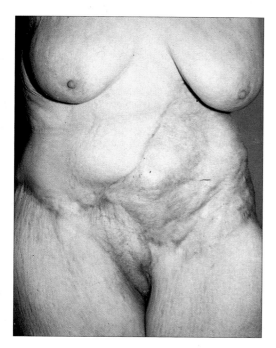

2.4 Necrotising fasciitis. Extensive debridement was required in the patient seen in **2.3** to prevent further spread of infection (*above*), and the resultant defect was managed by split-skin grafting which is shown fully covered three years later (*left*).

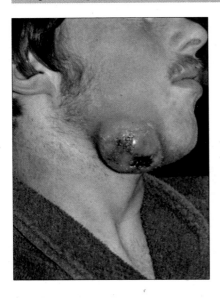

2.5 Disseminated tuberculosis.
Following a 3-month visit to India, this patient presented with a rapidly enlarging painful cervical mass on the right side of the neck, initially thought to be a large *Staphyloccocal* abscess. Incision and drainage of the abscess found pus and caseating lymph nodes. The diagnosis of secondary *Staphyloccocal* infection in tuberculous lymph nodes was based on both microscopy and Ziehl–Nielsen staining of abscess tissue which yielded *Staphyloccocal* organisms and alcohol- and acid-fast bacilli, and a 6-week culture for *Mycobacterium tuberculosis*. A chest radiograph confirmed a primary focus of infection in the apex of the right lung. Ziehl–Nielsen staining of sputum also yielded alcohol- and acid-fast bacilli. The systemic infection responded to prolonged anti-tuberculous chemotherapy.

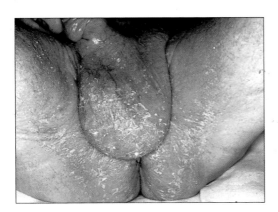

2.6 Perineal fungal infection. The patient had previously undergone anterior resection of the rectum and postoperative radiotherapy. This complication responded to treatment with an intravenous antifungal agent (fluconazole).

3.

BURNS

Burns are caused by dry (e.g. flame) or wet (e.g. hot liquid) heat. The extent and depth of the injury is dependent on the area and duration of contact. If inspection of the face demonstrates singeing of nostril hairs or evidence of pharyngitis, the clinician should have a high index of suspicion that there may be a concomitant inhalational injury. Arterial blood gases may indicate a high partial pressure of carbon monoxide.

Classification
• Superficial partial thickness.
• Deep partial thickness.
• Full thickness.

Full thickness skin grafts are required if it seems likely that contracture of a **split skin** graft could result in functional restriction (e.g. of the eyelids or the hands). **Composite free** or vascularised grafts may be required where muscle or periosteum have been injured, in order to attain coverage of the defect.

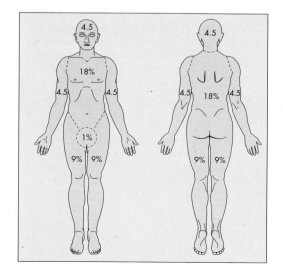

3.1 Body area percentages. For the purposes of resuscitation the 'rule of nines' is used to determine the extent of a burn injury. To calculate smaller areas, 1% of the body surface area is represented by the palmar surface of the patient's hand.

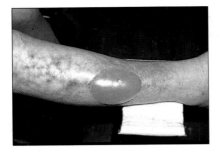

3.2 Superficial partial thickness burn.

This burn blister was caused by prolonged sitting in front of an electric fire. The elderly patient has peripheral vascular disease and displays **erythema ab igne** ('tinker's tartan'). Erythema caused by capillary dilatation and blistering by exudation of plasma beneath the coagulated epidermis is exquisitely painful. This injury was treated by leaving it exposed. As the germinal layer is intact, complete healing occurred within three weeks, with no residual scarring.

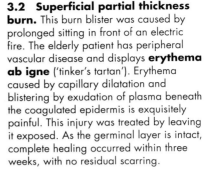

3.3 Deep partial thickness burn.

The injury was caused by a firework and left the germinal layer partially destroyed (deep dermal). There is intense blistering, followed by sloughing of the burnt area. As fewer epithelial elements survive, the attenuated surviving dermis heals with the production of disfiguring hypertrophic scars. While exposure of the burn is preferable, to allow the evaporation of protein-rich exudate, it is extremely difficult to manage burns effectively in this manner while preventing infection. This burn was dealt with by topical application of silver sulphadiazine cream and protection of the affected hand in a polythene bag.

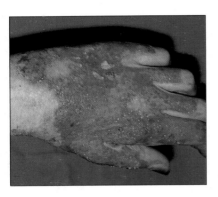

3.4 Deep partial thickness burn.

This injury resulted from a petrol burn. The degree of injury, involving the germinal layer, necessitated tangential excision, consisting of shaving away the outer, dead layers of skin down to the deep dermal layer. This was followed by skin grafting.

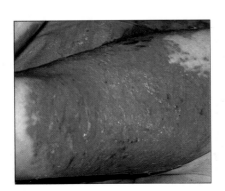

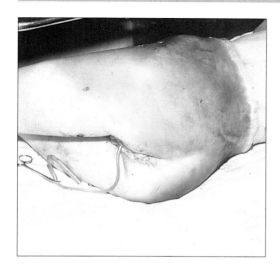

3.5 Full thickness burn.
This typical girdle-distribution injury was the result of flame burns from a nightdress which ignited as the patient stood in front of a gas fire. All layers of the skin are injured. If the extent of total burns is less than 10%, primary excision and immediate application of split-skin grafting can be undertaken. Where there is extensive burning and donor skin is limited, meshing the split skin graft can cover up to nine times the area, though in practice a ratio of three or four times the area is used, as the quality of the cosmetic result is more acceptable. Alternatives are temporary occlusive 'biological' dressings, which include porcine skin, amnion and stored homograft skin.

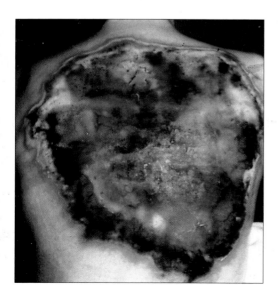

3.6 Eschar. Eschar-affected skin is insensate, and is woody or leathery on palpation. Escharotomy is necessary to release oedematous bands of constricting burned tissue, which may compromise respiration when the chest is involved and may compromise the circulation if the limbs are affected. Escharotomies are performed where possible along the axial lines of limbs.

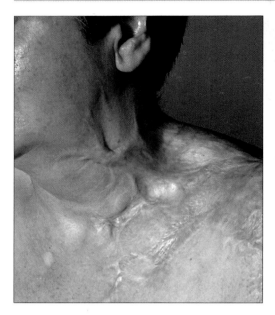

3.7 Hypertrophic keloid scar. This is the result of a healed deep dermal burn. Keloids can potentially occur in any wound, but dark-skinned races are more prone to develop hypertrophic scars than are Caucasians. Treatment is expectant, with the long-term application of pressure dressings and local steroid injections, if necessary. Re-excision of wounds only leads to further keloid formation.

4.

POSTOPERATIVE COMPLICATIONS

Any operation carries with it the risk of complications, and these may be related to the anaesthetic, the surgical intervention in general, or may be specifically related to the type of procedure undertaken.

These complications may involve the operation site itself (**local**) or they may affect any other system in the body (**general**). Postoperative complications can perhaps best be considered as being:

- **Immediate**: within the first few days of surgery.
- **Early**: within the first few weeks of surgery.
- **Late**: occurring at any subsequent time and often long after the surgical procedure has been undertaken.

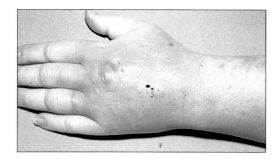

4.1 Phlebitis. This patient developed a postoperative pyrexia four days after surgery. A painful swelling was noted at the site of insertion of an intravenous cannula. There is obvious erythema and swelling.

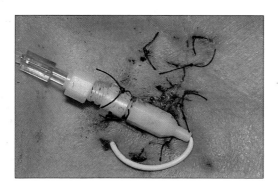

4.2 Central line (exit site infection). This patient underwent multiple inappropriate attempts at insertion of a central line for intravenous nutrition. Pus is exuding from the exit site. Cultures of the skin and blood grew *S. aureus*. The patient's pyrexia resolved when the line was removed.

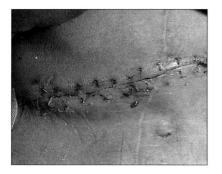

4.3   Wound infection. This patient's healing subcostal wound shows discharge of serous fluid on the eighth postoperative day. The patient had experienced an intermittent low-grade pyrexia in the post-operative period, following complex biliary surgery. A wound swab cultured *Escherichia coli*, but in the absence of significant systemic upset, antibiotic therapy was withheld and the patient's pyrexia resolved following the discharge of this fluid.

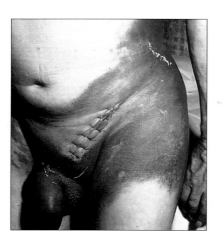

4.4   Wound haematoma. This patient developed swelling and bruising around the wound of a left inguinal hernia repair. These signs developed some five days after surgery, and almost certainly arose from reactionary haemorrhage from subcutaneous vessels. The patient had been on warfarin therapy for valvular heart disease.

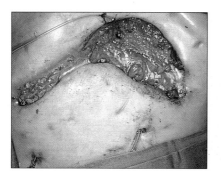

4.5   Wound dehiscence. The abdomen of a patient whose wound had disrupted on the seventh postoperative day. The patient had previously undergone an inappropriate attempt at resection of a bile duct tumour. The patient experienced an anastomotic leak which resulted in intra-abdominal sepsis. A history of chronic obstructive airways disease and long-term steroid therapy may have contributed to the subsequent wound dehiscence.

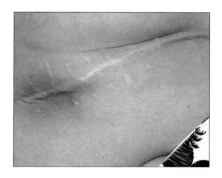

4.6 Late wound infection. The right subcostal scar of a patient who had previously undergone open cholecyst-ectomy. The patient developed a painful, hot swelling of the lateral extremity of the wound some five years following chole-cystectomy. Exploration of the wound demonstrated infection at the site of the knot of non-absorbable suture material.

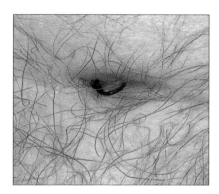

4.7 Stitch sinus. This complication arose 12 months after a recurrent right inguinal hernia repair. A multi-braided suture had been used in the repair. This has been managed conservatively by removal of the extruded suture material.

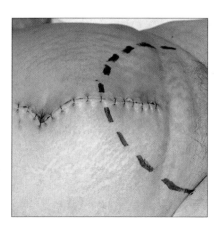

4.8 Urinary retention. The patient developed painless swelling of the lower abdomen on the first postoperative day following elective surgery. No urine had been passed since surgery and abdominal examination confirmed the presence of a distended palpable bladder which was dull to percussion. The bladder contained in excess of 1000 ml of urine following catheterisation.

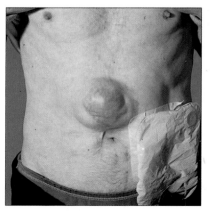

4.9 Incisional hernia. This patient had noted a progressive swelling at the site of a previous midline abdominal wound for revisional gastric surgery. The patient had always been able to reduce the swelling spontaneously through a broad-based defect measuring 12 cm in diameter. This incisional hernia was not repaired, since the patient was not at immediate risk of obtruction. Furthermore, a previous Hartman's resection had left the patient with a colostomy and it was felt that repair with prosthetic mesh would carry a substantial risk of infection.

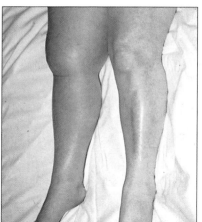

4.10 Deep vein thrombosis. This patient complained of a painful, tender, swollen calf one week following colectomy for inflammatory bowel disease. This had developed despite early mobilisation and subcutaneous heparin prophylaxis. Bilateral ascending venograms demonstrated the presence of clot in the deep femoral veins and accordingly the patient was heparinised and a compression stocking applied. The patient developed no further complications but was maintained on warfarin therapy for six months following the development of this complication.

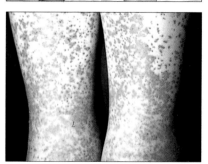

4.11 Drug hypersensitivity rash. This rash developed immediately following the administration of intravenous cephalosporin. This was managed by topical application of calamine lotion and oral antihistamine therapy.

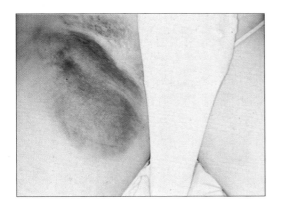

4.12 Haematoma after femoral artery puncture. Inadequate pressure on the arterial puncture site for blood gas analysis resulted in an immediate haematoma which steadily increased in size over the subsequent 30 minutes.

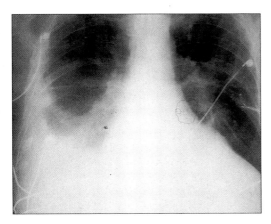

4.13 Pulmonary atelectasis with pleural effusion. This patient developed dypsnoea, tachycardia and mild pyrexia 48 hours after abdominal surgery. Examination confirmed dullness to percussion at the right base, and bronchial breath sounds on auscultation. The patient's symptoms, signs and chest radiograph improved with aggressive physiotherapy.

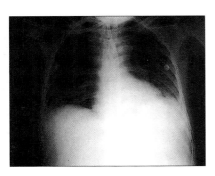

4.14 Left pleural effusion. This chest radiograph reveals opacification at the left base. The patient developed a swinging pyrexia 10 days after emergency splenectomy, and subsequently required percutaneous drainage of a left subphrenic abscess. The reactive pleural effusion cleared with drainage of the abscess.

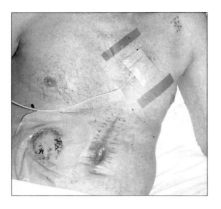

4.15 Duodenal fistula. An abdominal wound demonstrating discharge of purulent fluid from a drain site on the twelfth postoperative day.

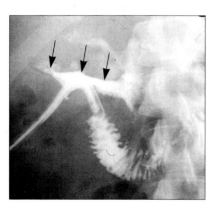

4.16 Duodenal fistula. Fistulogram demonstrating communication between wound and duodenal stump in a patient who has previously undergone a distal gastrectomy for recurrent peptic ulceration. The patient had no overt signs of sepsis and was managed by bowel rest and intravenous nutrition.

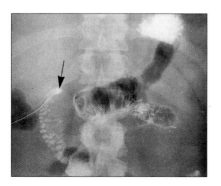

4.17 Duodenal fistula. Gastrograffin meal undertaken in the same patient as in **4.16** three weeks later demonstrated reflux from the gastric remnant into the duodenal loop. A small amount of contrast can be seen leaking from the duodenal stump but the fistula has almost completely healed on conservative therapy.

5.

NECK

When considering the **differential diagnosis** of a swelling in the neck it is important to determine the likely underlying tissue of origin, based on a basic knowledge of cervical anatomy and the investing layers binding the structures together.

Differential Diagnosis of a Neck Swelling

Skin and superficial fascia (See section 2)
- Sebaceous cyst.
- Sublingual dermoid.
- Lipoma.
- Other benign or malignant skin lesions.

Muscle
- Rhabdomyoma.
- Rhabdomyosarcoma.

Lymph nodes
- Reactive.
- Primary malignant.
- Infective.
- Secondary malignant.

Lymphatics
- Cystic hygroma.

Vascular
- Arteriovenous malformation.
- Subclavian/carotid artery aneurysm.
- Carotid body tumour.

Salivary glands (See section 3)
- Submandibular tumour.
- Parotid tumour.
- Sialectasis.
- Parotitis.

Pharynx (See section 3)
- Pharyngeal pouch.

Larynx
- Laryngocele.

Embryological
- Branchial cyst/fistula.
- Thyroglossal cyst.

Skeletal
- Cervical rib.

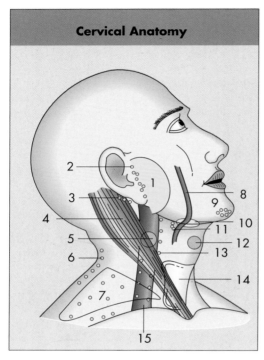

Cervical Anatomy

1 Parotid
2 Pre-auricular lymph nodes
3 Post-auricular lymph nodes
4 Sternocleidomastoid
5 Branchial cyst
6 Occipital lymph nodes
7 Supraclavicular lymph nodes
8 Facial artery
9 Submental lymph nodes
10 Submandibular gland
11 Submandibular lymph nodes
12 Thyroglossal cyst
13 Deep cervical chain of lymph nodes
14 Thyroid
15 Internal jugular vein

5.1   Diagrammatic illustration of the neck. The neck is broadly divided into anterior and posterior triangles by the sternocleidomastoid muscle, an easily recognised landmark, bounded anteriorly by the midline and posteriorly by the line of the trapezius.

Examination and Characteristics of a Neck Swelling

Irrespective of the site of a swelling, the principles of inspection, palpation and auscultation can be applied in order to formulate a **differential diagnosis**.

Inspection: Site, overlying skin colour, presence of skin tethering, *peau d'orange* infiltration, ulceration.

Palpation: Tenderness, skin temperature, size, surface texture, borders, solid/cystic, consistency, superficial/deep fixity, transillumination, regional lymphatic drainage, vascular thrill, pulsatility.

Auscultation: Bruit.

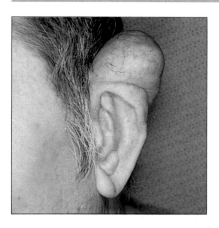

5.2 Sebaceous cyst. Situated behind the ear, the cyst is adherent to the skin and freely mobile over bone. Infection is common in these cysts and, if not fully excised, recurrence is likely.

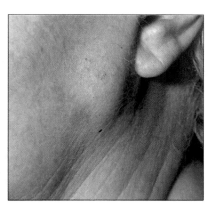

5.3 Lymphadenopathy. A painless and hard jugulo–digastric lymph node at the angle of the mandible. This patient was shown to have tonsillar carcinoma. The principal **differential diagnosis** is that of a parotid swelling.

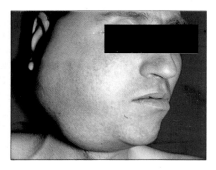

5.4 Lymphadenopathy. Mass of nodes (deep upper cervical chain) in the anterior triangle of the neck in a middle-aged man with metastatic melanoma which was confirmed by fine-needle aspiration cytology.

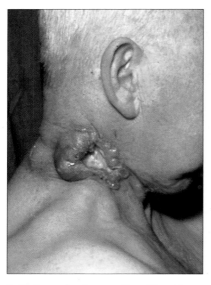

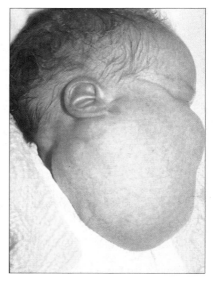

5.5 Lymphadenopathy. Ulcerating mass of malignant lymph nodes from a primary squamous cell carcinoma of the tongue.

5.6 Cystic hygroma. The majority of these appear at birth and usually affect the neck and axilla. Surgical excision is the only successful treatment and may be required as an emergency if the airway is obstructed. Excision is technically difficult due to the intimate involvement of the major nerves and vessels and, unless excision is complete, local recurrence is common. Sclerotherapy has been used to treat recurrent swellings.

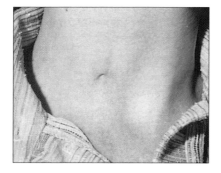

5.7 Branchial fistula. This shows a fistulous opening onto the neck which intermittently discharges mucus, without branchial cyst formation, and communicates upwards between the internal and external carotid arteries with the pharynx. Alternatively it may open into the tonsillar fossa. The whole tract must be dissected from skin to pharynx, otherwise the fistula will recur.

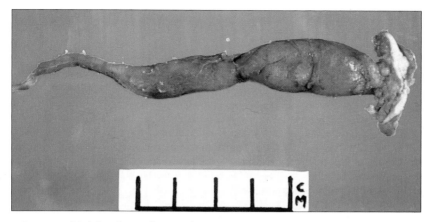

5.8 Branchial fistula and cyst. The pathological specimen illustrates the cutaneous exit of the fistula, the underlying cyst and the fistulous tract which was resected into the pharynx. This lesion arises from the second branchial arch and the swelling is positioned on the anterior border of the sternocleidomastoid at the junction of its upper and lower two thirds. If the cyst becomes infected the differential diagnosis then includes acute lymphadenitis or tuberculosis. Squamous epithelium lines the cyst which contains cholesterol crystals. These can be aspirated and examined by polarising microscopy which is diagnostic.

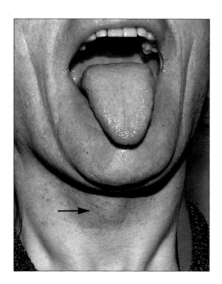

5.9 Thyroglossal cyst. This midline swelling (arrow) is attached to the foramen caecum in the posterior third of the tongue and the back of the hyoid bone. The cyst characteristically moves superiorly when the tongue is protruded because of the associated tract, which must be excised with the cyst. The **differential diagnosis** includes thyroid isthmus swellings which do not move with protrusion of the tongue.

6.

Breast

Understanding the lymphatic drainage of the breast is important as it has implications for the spread of **malignant disease** and its treatment.

The **cardinal symptoms and signs** of breast disease are a breast mass, pain, change in shape of the breast, scaling or **eczema of the nipple** and abnormal discharge from the nipple. The factors in the history which are important in relation to risk of breast cancer are parity, age at first pregnancy, menopausal status, hormone replacement therapy, smoking, previous history of **breast disease** and family history of **breast cancer**.

Principal Differential Diagnosis of a Swelling in the Breast
- Localised benign nodularity.
- Fibroadenoma.
- Carcinoma.
- Cyst.
- Breast abscess.
- Periductal mastitis/duct ectasia.

Other Differential Diagnosis
- Fat necrosis.
- Galactocele.
- Benign tumours – duct papilloma
                  – lipoma.

Diagnosis
- Clinical examination of both breasts, axillary and cervical lymph nodes.
- General examination.
- Mammography.
- Breast ultrasonography.
- Fine-needle aspiration cytology.
- Trucut biopsy.
- Excision biopsy.

Diagnosis in most lesions in the breast can be determined by a combination of clinical examination, imaging (mammography in the over-35 age group, ultrasound in the under-35 age group) and fine-needle aspiration cytology.

Levels of Axillary Nodes

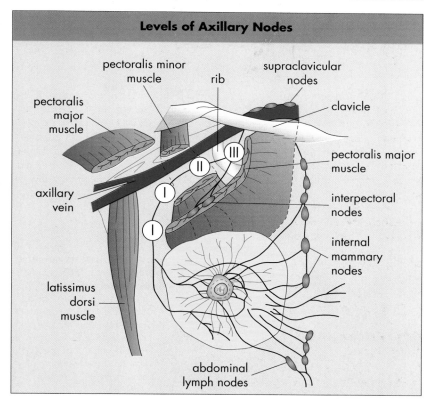

6.1 The majority of the lymphatic drainage from the breast is via the axillary and internal mammary nodes. The axillary nodes receive approximately 75% of the total lymph drainage and this is reflected in a greater frequency of tumour metastases to these nodes. Axillary nodes which are found below the axillary vein can be divided into three groups in relation to pectoralis minor muscle: Level 1 lies lateral to the pectoralis minor; Level 2 (central) nodes lie behind the pectoralis minor; and Level 3 (apical) nodes lie between the medial border of the pectoralis minor muscle, the first rib and axillary vein. There are, on average, twenty nodes in the axilla with approximately thirteen nodes at Level 1, five nodes at Level 2 and two at Level 3. Prognosis in breast cancer relates both to the number and level of axillary nodes involved.

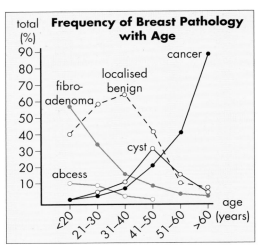

Frequency of Breast Pathology with Age

total (%)

90
80
70 — fibro-
60 — adenoma
50
40
30 — cyst
20
10 — abcess

localised benign

cancer

age (years)

<20 21-30 31-40 41-50 51-60 >60

6.2 Frequency of breast pathology with age.

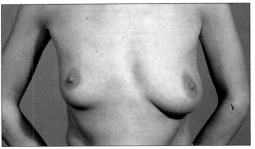

6.3 Normal asymmetry.
Most women's breasts are of an unequal size, but sometimes this difference is accentuated. The left breast is usually the larger. If clinical examination is normal and mammograms, if appropriate, show no discrete abnormality then the patient is simply reassured.

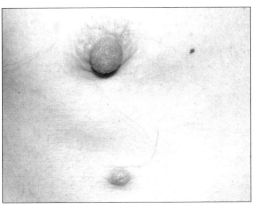

6.4 Accessory nipple.
Between 1–4% of women have an accessory nipple running in the milk-line from the axilla to the groin. The most common position for an accessory nipple is below the breast and above the umbilicus. Usually reassurance is all that is required, but if it is cosmetically unacceptable it can be excised under local anaesthesia.

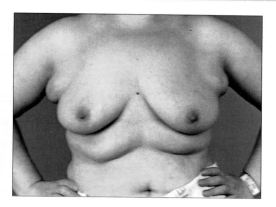

6.5 Accessory breast tissue. The most common site for the accessory breast is in the axilla. This woman has bilateral accessory axillary breasts. These had been causing her considerable embarrassment over a number of years and were treated by excision.

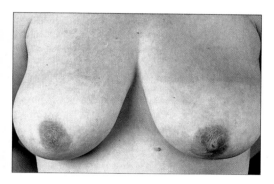

6.6 Bilateral eczema of the nipple. This patient presented with dry, scaly excoriation of both areolar regions. The main **differential diagnosis** is Paget's disease, which is principally unilateral and always involves the nipple. In contrast, the eczema usually starts in the areola and spreads to the nipple. This patient responded to topical hydrocortisone cream.

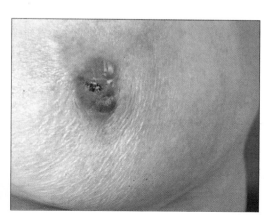

6.7 Paget's disease. This is an eczematous condition of the nipple/areolar complex. In its early stages (as shown) changes in the nipple are subtle. Approximately 1–2% of patients with breast cancer have Paget's disease. In 50% it is associated with underlying mass lesion. This lesion should be differentiated from eczema of the nipple and from direct spread into the nipple by an adjacent invasive carcinoma as shown in **6.10.**

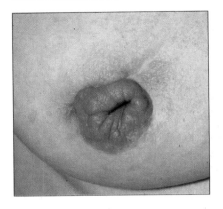

6.8 Nipple inversion due to periductal mastitis. This condition affects young women and is thought to be a smoking-related disease. The photograph demonstrates erythema around the nipple and the scars of multiple previous operations. She was treated with Augmentin and subsequently underwent further surgery including a total duct excision and nipple eversion.

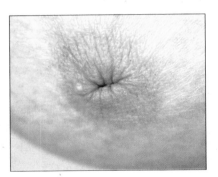

6.9 Nipple inversion due to duct ectasia. This condition is age-related and as women age, the ducts characteristically shorten and dilate, resulting in inversion, which is characteristically slit-like as seen here. This inversion should be clearly separated from that seen in malignant disease where the whole of the nipple is characteristically pulled in, as shown in **6.10**.

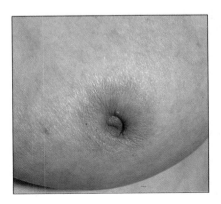

6.10 Nipple inversion in malignant disease.

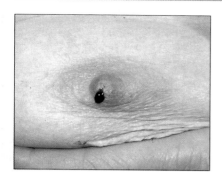

6.11 Nipple discharge. This elderly patient presented with a short history of a spontaneous single-duct blood-stained nipple discharge. Causes of blood-stained nipple discharge are duct papilloma, carcinoma *in situ* and duct ectasia. The most common cause of non-blood-stained nipple discharge is physiological discharge. This characteristically varies in colour from white, yellow, green or blue to black and is rarely spontaneous. Nipple discharge which is not frankly blood-stained should be tested for blood using a dipstix. Persistent, troublesome or bloody discharges (overt or only detected on stix testing) require further investigation.

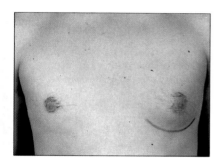

6.12 Gynaecomastia. This 13-year-old boy presented with tender enlargement of the left breast. It commonly occurs at puberty and is seen in 30–60% of boys. It usually requires no treatment as 80% resolve spontaneously. Rarely, as shown here, the asymmetry is marked and surgery is required.

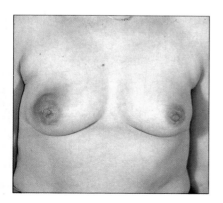

6.13 Non-lactational breast abscess. Abscesses in the breast are now less common than they used to be. And non-lactational breast abscesses, usually occurring in the peri-areolar region are now more common than lactational abscesses. The organisms responsible for non-lactational infection are usually a combination of anaerobes and aerobes.

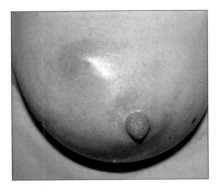

6.14 Lactational abscess. These usually occur within the first few weeks of breast feeding and are characteristically due to *Staphylococcus aureus*. Most breast abscesses (lactational or non-lactational) can be treated by the application of local anaesthetic cream left *in situ* for 1 hour, followed by aspiration repeated every 2–3 days and combined with appropriate oral antibiotic therapy or mini-incision, drainage and regular daily irrigation with saline.

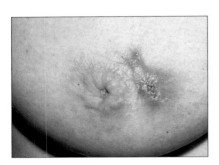

6.15 Mammary duct fistula. This condition is a complication of periductal mastitis. This patient had recurrent episodes of peri-areolar infection and abscess formation; and, following incision and drainage of a non-lactational abscess, developed a fistula which persisted despite attempts at fistula excision. She was subsequently referred to a specialist breast unit, where re-excision of the fistula was combined with a total duct excision and nipple eversion. The wound was primarily closed and the operation, carried out under antibiotic cover with Augmentin, was successful.

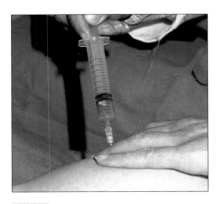

6.16 Breast cysts. This patient had a previous history of breast cysts and presented with a clearly defined breast mass which proved to be cystic on aspiration.

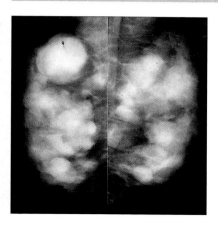

6.17 Mammogram of cystic disease. Multiple bilateral haloed opacities are visible in both breasts.

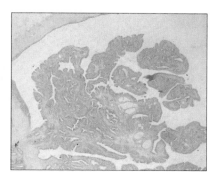

6.18 Intraduct papilloma. This patient presented with a serous nipple discharge and the histological specimen showed an intraduct papilloma with a fibrovascular core lined by columnar epithelium.

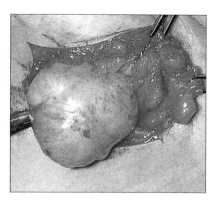

6.19 Fibroadenoma. These are no longer considered to be benign tumours but to be aberrations of normal breast development. They are most common (**6.2**) in women below the age of 35. Few fibroadenomas increase in size and a diagnosis of fibroadenoma can be made by a combination of clinical examination, fine-needle aspiration cytology and ultrasound.

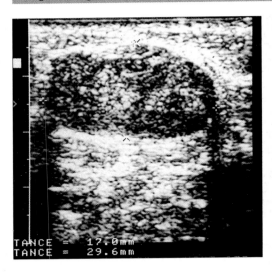

6.20 Ultrasonogram of a fibroadenoma. A well-demarcated lesion with clear margins is seen.

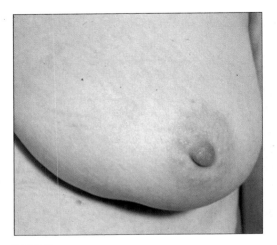

6.21 Carcinoma of breast. This 65-year-old noticed a change in contour of her left breast. Skin dimpling was evident in the lower inner quadrant of the left breast, a feature characteristic of breast cancer.

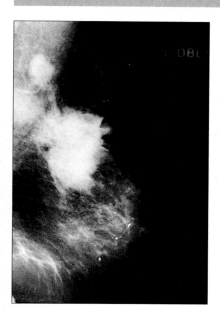

6.22 Mammography of a breast carcinoma. This mammogram shows a large irregular spiculated mass lesion in the upper outer quadrant of the left breast associated with an enlarged pathological node in the left axilla. These features are characteristic of a breast carcinoma associated with axillary node metastases.

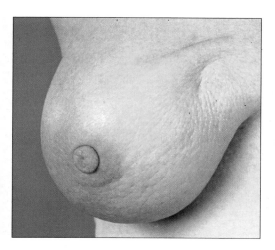

6.23 *Peau d'orange.* This is a sign of locally advanced breast cancer and can be accentuated by finger pressure. The appearances are due to lymphatic oedema caused by malignant lymphatic infiltration. The pits represent the fixed opening of the sweat ducts which cannot expand with the oedema. Initial treatment of these patients is by a primary systemic therapy followed either by radiotherapy or surgery.

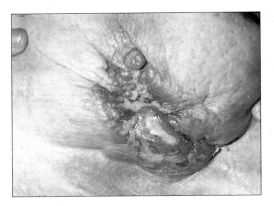

6.24 Ulcerated carcinoma of the breast.

This elderly patient had had an ulcerating lesion of her breast for 9 months prior to presentation. Initial treatment was directed at wound toilet. Thereafter she received treatment with tamoxifen and radiotherapy.

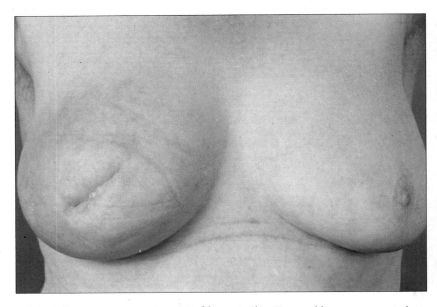

6.25 Inflammatory carcinoma of breast. This 45-year-old women presented with a one-month history of pain and swelling of the right breast. She was initially treated with antibiotics but this failed to resolve. Clinically, she had a large carcinoma associated with palpable clinically involved axillary lymph node. The lesion was treated by primary systemic chemotherapy with a good response.

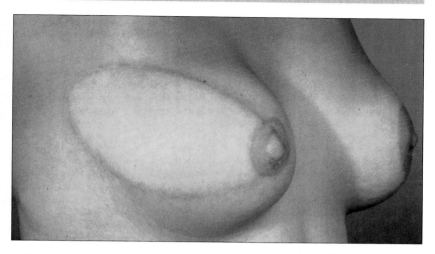

6.26 Latissimus dorsi flap reconstruction. This 26-year-old had a 3 cm invasive carcinoma of the right breast associated with widespread surrounding *in situ* disease. She was treated with mastectomy and latissimus dorsi flap reconstruction. She later underwent nipple-areolar reconstruction. Although the major bulk of the reconstructed breast is due to the latissimus dorsi muscle, a silicone prosthesis was inserted beneath the muscle to produce symmetry.

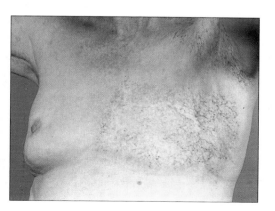

6.27 Radiodermatitis. This patient had undergone mastectomy and axillary node sampling, followed by radiotherapy to the chest wall and axilla 15 years earlier. There are characteristic changes of telangiectasia, which is associated with skin damage by radiotherapy.

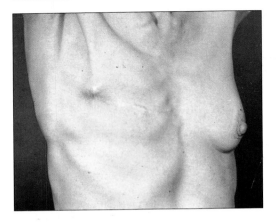

6.28 Recurrent carcinoma of breast. This patient had had a mastectomy 15 years previously and developed a nodule in the mastectomy scar, which on investigation was shown to be recurrent carcinoma.

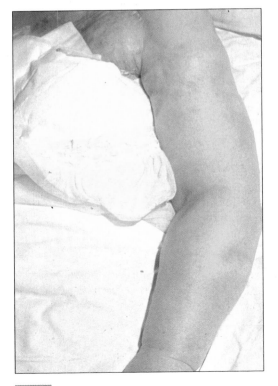

6.29 Lymphoedema. This patient, presenting with lymphoedema, had been treated previously for carcinoma of the left breast by a mastectomy, axillary node sampling and postoperative radiotherapy to the breast and axilla. Lymphoedema can follow either surgery or radiotherapy alone, but is most commonly seen when extensive surgery and radiotherapy are combined. It can also develop in association with axillary recurrence. Lymphoedema is difficult to treat and a combination of bandaging, a pressure graduated stocking and regular use of extrinsic compression pumps are often required to improve symptoms.

Section 2

Skin, its Adnexae and Subcutaneous Tissue

7.

BENIGN CONDITIONS

Diagnosis

To reach a definitive diagnosis of a skin swelling, the examination should determine whether the lesion is:

- Located in the skin or subcutaneous tissue.
- Epidermal or dermal.
- Pigmented.

Skin or subcutaneous tissue

This may be determined by pinching the skin over the swelling and attempting to move it from side to side. If the swelling is in the skin, neither can be moved independently.

Epidermal or dermal

The stretched, normal epithelium overlying a dermal swelling may look glossy but normally remains smooth. Ulceration may result from pressure necrosis if the swelling is large. An epithelial lesion causes roughening of the skin surface, papilliform growth or ulceration, even when it is of small size.

Pigmented

Melanin produces black or brown pigmentation, while haemosiderin produces brown or yellow pigmentation. In general, melanin pigmentation is characteristic of melanocytic activity, but certain other skin lesions (for example, basal cell carcinoma or seborrhoeic keratosis) may show melanin pigmentation.

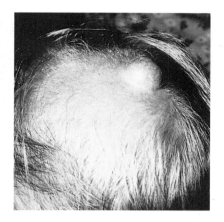

7.1   Sebaceous cyst. Such lesions have thin walls of flattened epidermal cells and contain a cheesy white material composed of epithelial debris and sebum having a characteristic, sweet, musty smell. They are found on hair-bearing areas such as the scalp, face, ears, neck, back and scrotum. These hemispherical smooth soft swellings lie within the skin. The overlying epithelium is normal but a small punctum, marking the site of the involved hair follicle, is common.

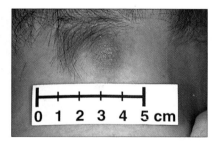

7.2   Infected sebaceous cyst. Excision of the cyst under local anaesthesia is all that is required unless the cyst becomes infected, in which case simple incision and drainage should be undertaken if there is a failed response to antibiotics, followed by secondary excision at a later date.

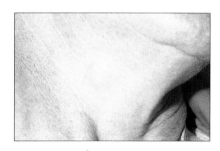

7.3   Dermoid cyst. This is a subcutaneous cystic swelling commonly found on the fingers. These may occur as an embryological anomaly or as an implantation of epidermoid cells from the skin as the result of a puncture. The cyst is lined by squamous epithelium and contains sebum, degenerate cells and, sometimes, hair. The cyst may be fixed deeply, particularly when situated on the face or neck as shown here. Implantation dermoids may be removed under local anaesthesia, whereas congenital cysts may extend more deeply and require formal dissection under general anaesthesia.

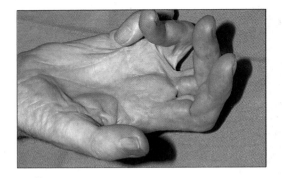

7.4 Dupuytren's contracture. This condition results from thickening and contracture of either the palmar or plantar aponeurosis, causing progressive flexion of the affected digits. The first sign is usually a small fibrous nodule or cord just distal to the distal palmar crease in the line of the fourth finger. This eventually causes a hook-like deformity as shown here. The aetiology is obscure but in some cases there is a familial history. Phenytoin ingestion, alcohol abuse or chronic ill-health may also be precipitating factors.

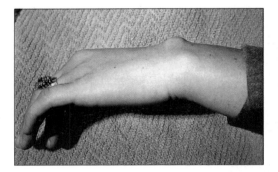

7.5 Ganglion of the wrist. This represents a benign myxoma of the joint capsule or tendon sheath and may be found around the wrist, on the dorsum of the foot, or the flexor aspect of the fingers and on the peroneal tendons. These ganglia are unilocular, thin-walled cysts with a synovial lining containing mucoid fluid. If they are asymptomatic and do not interfere with the function of the limbs, then no treatment is required. If this is not the case, then surgical excision with dissection of the lesion to its origin from the joint or tendon is required, with ligation of its neck.

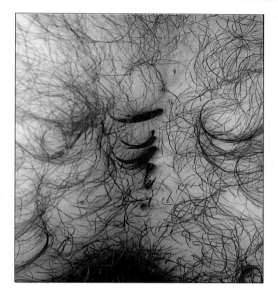

7.6 Pilonidal sinus. This post-natal cleft sinus exhibits the classical features of hair protruding from the sinus tracts. This patient is typical of the young male adult with dark hair who is susceptible to develop such sinuses. They may also be found in the clefts between the fingers (an occupational disease of barbers and hairdressers), and rarely in the axilla, umbilicus, perineum and the sole of the foot, as well as on amputation stumps. Infection and lateral extension of sinus tracts are common. The lesion is excised down to the post-sacral fascia and closed primarily in layers.

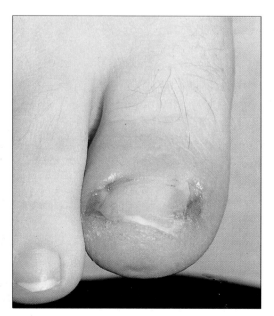

7.7 Ingrowing toenail. This is one of the most common conditions affecting young adults. Attendant morbidity is high. Infection and inflammation are common. Failure of chiropody is an indication of surgery. Ingrowing toenails are best treated by nail edge excision and phenolisation, or by excision of the nail bed.

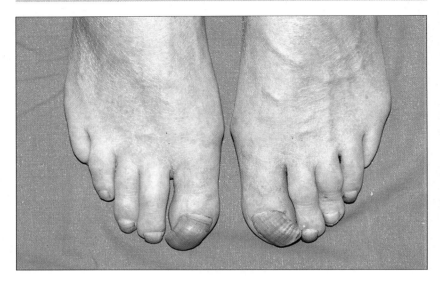

7.8 Onychogryphosis. The hallux is the most common site affected and the nail deformity is seen as a 'ram's horn'. It may follow trauma to the nail bed and is usually found in elderly subjects. Simple avulsion under digital block anaesthesia gives symptomatic relief but will invariably lead to recurrence. Symptomatic recurrences are an indication of definitive nail bed surgery.

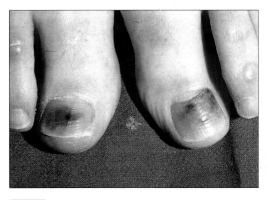

7.9 Subungual haematoma. This is the result of a crush injury to the terminal phalanx, with or without fracture to the under-lying bone. The intense pain can be relieved by evacuating the clot, either by using a dental drill or a red-hot needle. It is important to differentiate the condition from subungual melanoma (**8.30**).

8.

BENIGN AND MALIGNANT TUMOURS

Classification

Benign
- Papilloma.
- Verruca vulgaris.
- Dermatofibroma.
- Benign melanoma.
- Lipoma.
- Seborrhoeic keratosis.
- Keratoacanthoma.
- Haemangioma.
- Neurofibroma.

Premalignant
- Bowen's Disease.
- Chronic cutaneous ulceration.
- Solar keratosis.
- Lentigo maligna.
- Radiodermatitis.

Malignant
- Squamous cell carcinoma.
- Fibrosarcoma.
- Kaposi's sarcoma.
- Malignant melanoma.
- Basal cell carcinoma.
- Rhabdomyosarcoma.
- Metastases.

Cutaneous manifestations of malignancy
- Acanthosis nigrans.
- Lip pigmentation.
- Herpes zoster.
- Erythroderma.
- Pemphigoid.
- Dermatomyositis.
- Carcinoid facies.
- Finger clubbing.

Treatment is directed at surgical excision of the lesion, usually under local anaesthesia. As a general rule, malignant lesions require wider-margin excision, with or without primary closure or skin coverage with skin graft.

BENIGN TUMOURS AND HAMARTOMAS

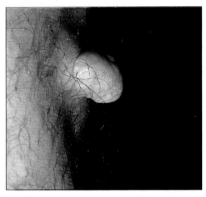

8.1 Pedunculated papilloma. These can occur at any site and form flesh coloured, spherical, warty masses which hang on a stalk of surrounding normal epithelium.

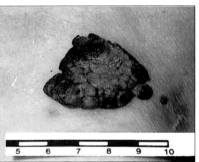

8.2 Seborrhoeic keratosis. This is a basal cell papilloma common in the elderly. It forms a yellowish, brown or black greasy plaque with a cracked surface which falls off in pieces, and has been likened to the end of a dirty paintbrush. They are often multiple, occurring particularly on the back and trunk.

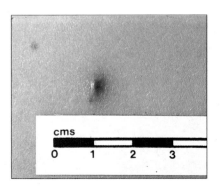

8.3 Dermatofibroma. This is a common fibrous tumour composed of histiocytes causing nodular subepithelial fibrosis, dealt with by simple excision.

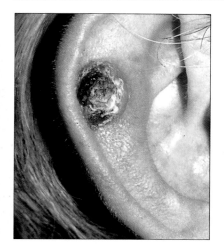 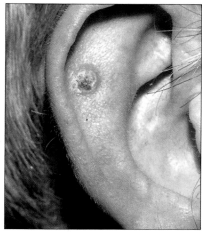

8.4 Keratoacanthoma. This lesion occurs most frequently on the face and nose
(75%), but may also be found on the fingers, hands and elsewhere on the skin of
patients of the 50- to 60-year-old age group. The rapidly growing nodule appears over a
few weeks and, if left untreated, will disappear over a 4–5 month period leaving a faint
white scar. The horn in this man's ear is shown at presentation (***left***), and four weeks
later with spontaneous regression (***right***). The principal **differential diagnosis** is that
of a squamous cell carcinoma and it is safest, therefore, to remove the lesion if only to
establish a histological diagnosis.

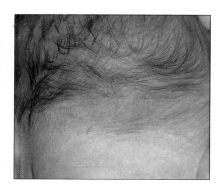

8.5 Capillary haemangioma. The
'port wine stain' is flat and varies in
colour from pink to bright red. It is present
at birth and does not regress with age. It
may be associated with similar lesions in
the nervous system.

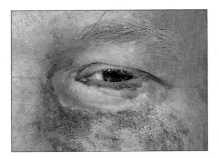

8.6 Capillary haemangioma. This can be a disfiguring malformation. This lesion has been partially treated successfully with a neodymium-YAG laser. Involvement of the lower eyelid necessitated use of a full-thickness skin graft. Appropriate application of make-up may also improve cosmetic appearance.

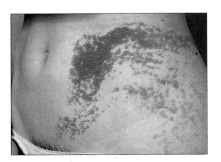

8.7 Cavernous haemangioma. This appears as a bluish-purple elevated mass which empties on pressure and slowly refills. Unlike the strawberry naevus, it does not appear until early childhood. Ulceration and bleeding may occur and can be serious, and therefore it is best treated by excision.

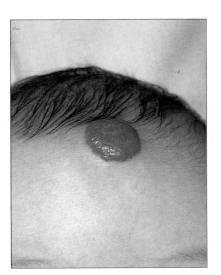

8.8 Strawberry naevus. The strawberry naevus usually appears at or within a few weeks of birth and predominantly affects the head and neck. Active growth continues for about 6 months but the lesion remains static until the child is 2–3 years of age, before it shrinks and loses its colour. It usually disappears before the child is 7 years of age and therefore the treatment is expectant rather than surgical.

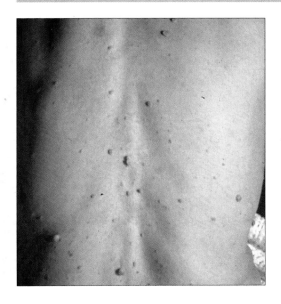

8.9 Neurofibroma. This is a hamartoma of neural tissue and may be solitary or multiple. If multiple (as shown), it may be associated with **von Recklinghausen's disease** (neurofibromatosis). This is a genetically transmitted autosomal disorder present at birth or becoming apparent in early childhood.

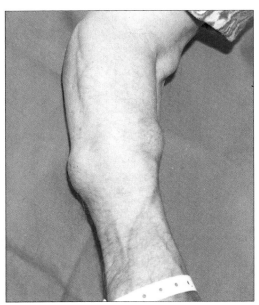

8.10 Lipoma. These lesions are frequently multiple, as shown on this patient's forearm. They are slow growing, benign tumours of fatty tissue which form a lobulated soft mass and are enclosed by a thin fibrous capsule. Sarcomatous change may occur in larger lipomas but is rare. Unless they are symptomatic or there is doubt about the diagnosis, lipomas do not usually require excision.

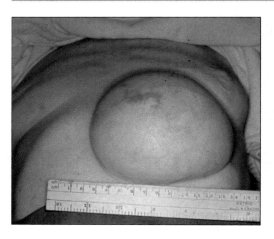

8.11 Giant lipoma and sarcomatous change.
If left untreated, lipomas can occasionally reach substantial size (as shown here). On examination, the lesion was soft and fluctuant, the overlying skin was freely mobile and the lobulation of the lesion was easily palpable. Excision confirmed the presence of a liposarcoma. Liposarcomas can also occur in the retroperitoneum.

BENIGN PIGMENTED MOLES

The pigment producing cells, **melanocytes**, lie in the basal layer of the epidermis. The number of melanocytes (approximately 2 million) is fixed, irrespective of the skin colour of the person, but the amount of pigment produced by them varies in individuals. A mole or **melanocytic naevus** is formed by an agglomeration of melanocytes which have migrated to the dermis or epidermis.

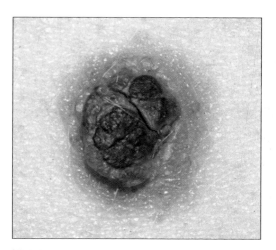

8.12 Melanocytic naevus. This lesion appears particularly on the face and trunk, especially around puberty. Macroscopically, it is a flat or slightly raised brown or black lesion covered by normal epidermis. Histologically, such lesions can be subdivided into dermal, junctional or compound naevi.

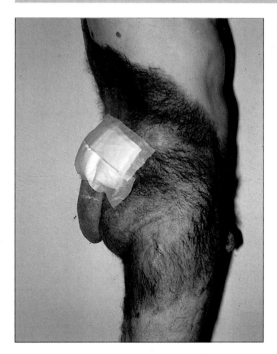

8.13 Giant hairy naevus. Unlike the melanocytic naevus, this congenital lesion is present at birth. It occupies a wide area which may correspond to a dermatome. In this patient, the extent is such that it is termed a 'bathing trunk naevus'.

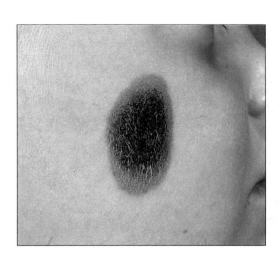

8.14 Giant hairy naevus. This 5-year-old girl had a cosmetically unacceptable hairy mole on the right side of face which was treated by sequential linear excision. Occasionally, larger naevi require split skin grafting.

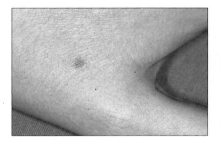

8.15   Blue naevus. This is a deep, intradermal naevus in which the blue colour is due to an optical effect caused by the depth of the lesion. It may develop at any time from birth to middle life and may form a blue-black papule on the face and arms, as a beauty spot, or as ribbon like areas on the wrist, ankle or buttock.

PREMALIGNANT SKIN CONDITIONS

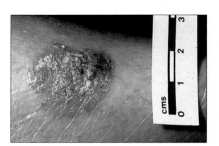

8.16   Bowen's disease. This intradermal condition appears as an area of brownish induration with a well defined edge, becoming nodular and forming a keratin crust as an intra-epidermal carcinoma develops.

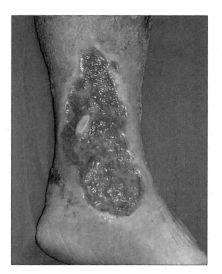

8.17   Chronic ulceration. This varicose ulcer, present for 12 years, had shown signs of recent extension and more pronounced crusting. Biopsy confirmed the presence of the development of a squamous cell carcinoma (**Marjolin's ulcer**).

MALIGNANT TUMOURS

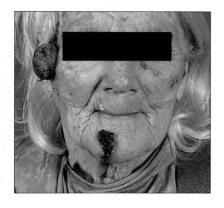

8.18 Squamous cell carcinoma.

This can occur anywhere on the surface of the body but is particularly common on exposed parts, i.e. the ears, cheeks, lower lips and the backs of the hands. This elderly woman with widespread actinic skin damage has two separate carcinomas of the face and chin. The predisposing factors include senile keratosis, Bowen's disease, lupus vulgaris, exposure to sunshine, radiation or carcinogens (pitch, tar, soot), and chronic ulceration.

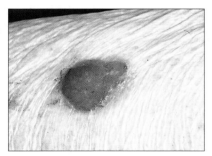

8.19 Squamous cell carcinoma.

The lesion starts as a hard, erythematous nodule which proliferates to form a cauliflower-like excrescence or ulcerates to form a malignant ulcer with a raised, fixed, hard edge. Metastasis to regional nodes occurs early in the disease and, in this patient, spread to the groin nodes.

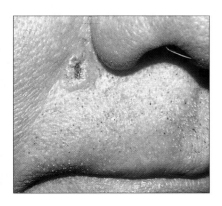

8.20 Basal cell carcinoma (rodent ulcer).

These lesions occur predominantly in the mid-portion of the face, especially in the nose, the inner canthus of the eye, the forehead and eyelids. They have a variable clinical appearance. This is a basal cell carcinoma affecting the nasolabial fold which was excised and the defect covered with an advancement flap.

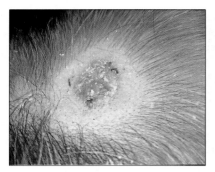

8.21   Ulcerated basal cell carcinoma. This lesion is situated on the vertex of the scalp and presented with bleeding.

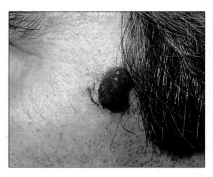

8.22   Cystic basal cell carcinoma. This variant bled profusely on minor trauma. Treatment is with primary excision, with or without skin grafting.

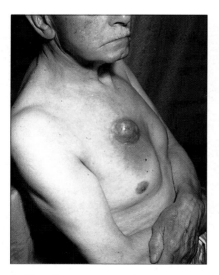

8.23   Fibrosarcoma. This tumour, arising from fibrous tissue, is most common in the lower limbs or buttocks but is shown here on the chest wall. It forms a large, deep and fixed mass surrounded by neovascularisation.

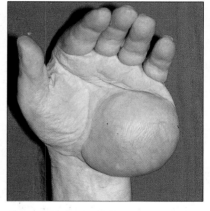

8.24   Rhabdomyosarcoma. This is a greyish-pink, soft, fleshy, lobulated well-circumscribed tumour arising from striated muscle, shown here arising from the hypothenar muscles. The tumour is more common in children, is highly malignant and requires treatment by radical excision or radiotherapy.

MALIGNANT MELANOMAS

Malignant melanomas predominantly affect Caucasians. The highest incidence in the world is in Queensland, Australia (17 per 100,000 population) and is a direct consequence of exposure to sunlight. Malignant melanomas constitute 3 per cent of malignant tumours of the skin, and approximately 50 per cent of malignant melanomas arise in **pre-existing naevi**. Although the risk of malignant change in a naevus is small, this risk is enhanced the greater number of naevi there are present. Although they are usually sited cutaneously, they can occur in the mucous membranes and the eye (conjunctiva, choroid, retina).

Signs of Malignant Change
- Increase in size.
- Increase in pigmentation.
- Bleeding or ulceration.
- Spread of pigment from edge of tumour.
- Itching or pain.
- Formation of daughter nodules.
- Lymph node or distant spread.

Classification
- Clark (according to depth of penetration).
- Breslow (actual thickness of the melanoma, measured in mm).

Treatment
- Wide excision.
- Regional lymph node block dissection.
- Radiotherapy.
- Regional chemotherapy.

There are **four distinct clinical pathological types** of malignant melanoma: lentigo maligna, superficial spreading, nodular and amelanotic variants.

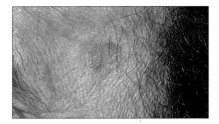

8.25 Lentigo maligna. Ten per cent of malignant melanomas arise in this lesion, which is otherwise known as the 'senile freckle'. The lesion shown here on this patient's left temple occurs most frequently on the face of elderly women, affecting particularly the lower eyelids, cheek, side of nose, forehead or neck. It is a brownish-red patch which grows slowly and centrifugally, and advances and recedes over many years. The edge of the lesion is serrated and map-like but the margin with normal skin is abrupt.

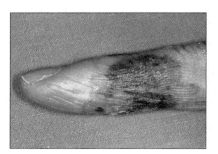

8.26 Superficial spreading melanoma. This is the most common variant of malignant melanoma, which occurs most frequently in middle age. It occurs predominantly on the trunk, although in this patient the lesion originates in the index finger. The surface of the lesion is slightly raised and its outline is indistinct. Pigmentation is patchy and there may be a wide range of colour. Digital amputation was carried out.

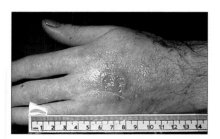

8.27 Amelanotic melanoma. Such melanomas are rare and are usually associated with rapid growth and lack of pigment, accounting for their pale pink colour.

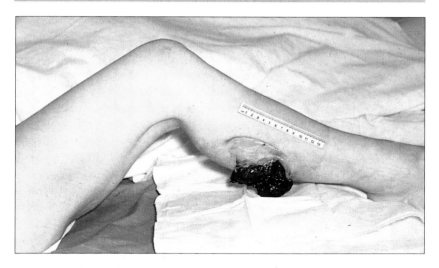

8.28 Nodular melanoma. This lesion on the right leg of a female patient is typical. It is vertically invasive and malignant from its onset. It starts as an elevated, deeply pigmented nodule which steadily enlarges both on the surface and by centrifugal extension. It progressively darkens and the surface over the area of active growth becomes jet black and glossy. Bleeding, crusting, scab formation, ulceration, itching and irritation are common.

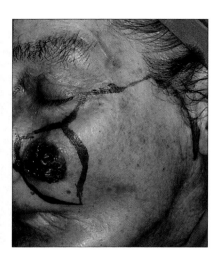

8.29 Nodular melanoma. Wide excision of this melanoma was undertaken and the defect covered by rotating a facial skin flap.

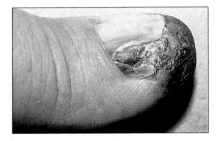

8.30 Subungual melanoma. This can occur in middle-aged and elderly patients. It affects the thumb or great toe where it may cause chronic inflammation below the nail. In this age group, it is often misdiagnosed as a subungual haematoma or an ingrowing toenail. (Reproduced with permission from White, *Colour Atlas of Regional Dermatology*, Mosby–Wolfe, 1994.)

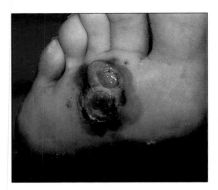

8.31 Plantar acral melanoma. Melanomas are rare in non-Caucasians, but where they do occur they are usually of this type.

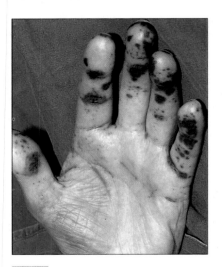

8.32 Metastatic melanoma. Multiple peripheral metastatic lesions are present in this patient's hand.

SKIN CHANGES ASSOCIATED WITH SYSTEMIC MALIGNANCY

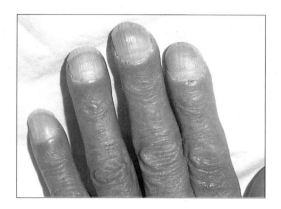

8.33 Finger clubbing.
This is a non-specific sign of a variety of benign and malignant systemic illnesses. It must be differentiated from familial finger clubbing.

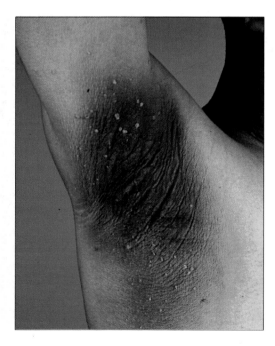

8.34 Acanthosis nigrans. The darkening of the skin on the flexural areas of the body is shown here in a patient with carcinoma of the stomach, producing thick, darkened and roughened skin.

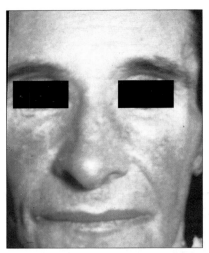

8.35 Carcinoid flush.

This is part of the carcinoid syndrome whereby excessive amounts of 5-hydroxy-tryptamine escape into the systemic circulation from a carcinoid tumour, usually of the small bowel with substantial metastatic disease in the liver, whereby the serotonin is usually metabolised. This results in flushing of the face, bronchospasm, tricuspid incompetence and diarrhoea.

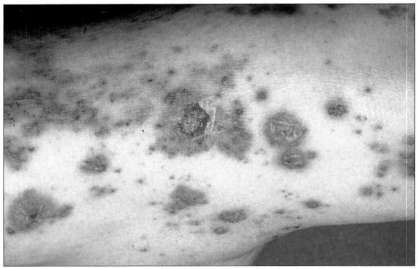

8.36 Herpes zoster. This 48-year-old heavy smoker presented initially with severe leg pain and a suspected lower limb fracture. Plain radiology was normal and the typical dermatome skin rash of zoster erupted 48 hours after admission. Chest radiography demonstrated a large bronchial neoplasm.

Section 3

Oromaxillofacial

9.

FACIAL FRACTURES

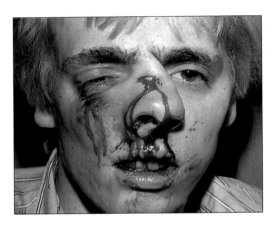

9.1 Fractured nose. This is a common injury which causes pain, swelling and tenderness over the root of the nose. Lateral blows tend to displace the nose to the contralateral side, as shown. Anterior trauma tends to result in nasal bridge depression and widening of the inner canthal distance. Periorbital haematoma and medial conjunctival haemorrhage are common findings. Epistaxis is present and bilateral. Deviation of the nose or injury to the septum requires early manipulation. Septal haematomas require urgent drainage to prevent cartilage necrosis.

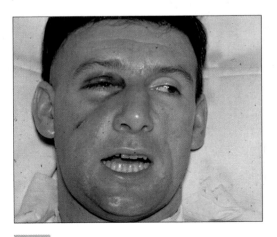

9.2 Fractured zygoma (malar fracture). This patient sustained a blow to the face which fractured the zygoma. Clinical features include periorbital haematoma, subconjunctival haemorrhage, a lack of normal cheek prominence due to zygomatic depression, unilateral epistaxis, limitation of mandibular movements and infraorbital paraesthesia. Palpation may reveal an infraorbital step.

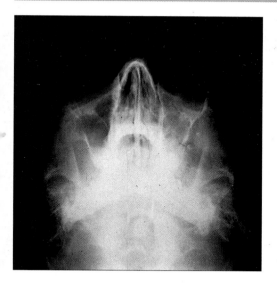

9.3 Fractured left zygoma. This occipito-mental radiograph shows a zygomatic fracture caused by a blow to the face. There are three fracture sites visible: at the fronto-zygomatic suture; on the zygomatic arch; and adjacent to the zygomatico-maxillary suture in relation to the infraorbital foramen. The antrum is opaque as it contains blood.

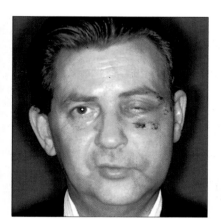
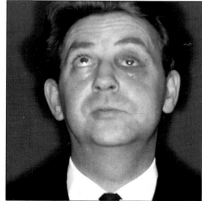

9.4 Fractured orbital floor. The rim of the orbit has been hit by a cricket ball causing an increase in orbital pressure and resulting in an orbital blow-out fracture (**left**). The patient presented with a disturbance of eye movements with tethering of the inferior rectus and oblique muscles by entrapment and herniation of the surrounding orbital fat. This is seen as resultant diplopia in the upward gaze (**right**).

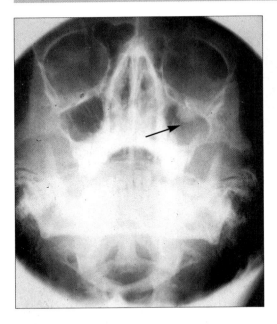

9.5 Fractured orbital floor. This radiograph shows herniation of the orbital contents into the antrum. There may be a substantial degree of prolapse into the antrum with trapping of the periorbital fat and fixing of the inferior rectus and oblique muscles preventing upward gaze. Fat atrophy and scarring may produce permanent enophthalmos and diplopia, even after treatment.

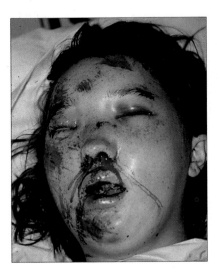

9.6 Central mid-face fracture. This patient sustained a mid-third facial fracture as a result of a road traffic accident. Her face hit the dashboard at high speed, resulting in a typical 'dish face' deformity with the central middle third of the face being displaced posteriorly along the base of skull. The cribriform plate was damaged, resulting in a cerebrospinal fluid rhinorrhoea.

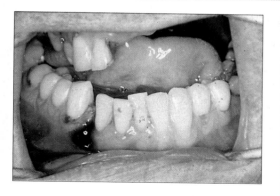

9.7 Fractured mandible.
This patient was involved in a fight, sustaining a fracture to the body of the mandible with localised soft tissue swelling. He was unable to close his teeth in occlusion and had impaired sensation to his lower lip due to disruption of the inferior alveolar nerve. Inspection of his mouth shows a localised sublingual haematoma which is pathognomonic of mandibular fracture.

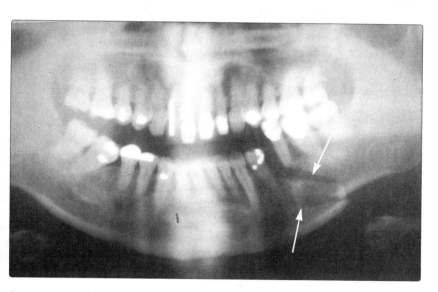

9.8 Fractured mandible. This panoral radiograph demonstrates the mandibular fractures and their degree and direction of displacement. Displaced mandibular fractures are usually fixed internally, with early return of function.

10.

ORAL CAVITY

The **mouth** is the most proximal part of the gastrointestinal tract, and thus forms an **essential part of the general examination**. The most common **symptoms** patients will present with are pain, swelling, ulceration, discharge, or loss of function making eating or swallowing difficult. Inflammatory lesions are usually painful, while early malignant disease may not be.

Inspection: the mouth should be examined with a pen torch and spatula, noting the state of the dentition and periodontium. Then all the soft tissues should be examined for abnormalities on the tongue, floor of the mouth, buccal mucosa, tonsillar fossae, palate and oropharynx.

The incidence and mortality rates of **malignant disease** of the mouth have increased since the 1970s, with a more marked increase in the younger age groups. Oral cancer is twice as common in males than females, and death is three times as likely in social class V compared with social class I. **Survival rates** for oral cancer vary across different anatomical sites, the prognosis for oropharyngeal cancer being poor in contrast to cancer of the upper alveolus. The overall rate, however, is less good than for more common cancers of the breast, cervix and colon. Although **95 per cent** of neoplastic lesions are **squamous cell carcinomas**, others include lymphomas and mucoepidermoid, adenoid-cystic and adeno-carcinomas of major or minor salivary glands.

Predisposing Factors to Malignancy

Chronic irritation
- Tobacco products for smoking and chewing.
- Spices.
- Ultra-violet light.
- Heavy alcohol consumption.

- Sepsis.

- Betel quid chewing in Asian populations.
- Ill-fitting dentures.
- Dental caries.

Miscellaneous
- Immunosuppression.

- Poor diet and nutrition.

Leukoplakia
Worldwide, 4 per cent of intraoral leukoplakias (white patches that do not rub off and cannot be attributed to a known cause) are said to show malignant change, whilst at least 50 per cent of the erythroplakias (red patches) may do so.

Iron deficiency

Plummer–Vinson syndrome, sideropaenic dysphagia in women characterised by glossitis, angular cheilitis and dysphagia, is associated with post-cricoid carcinoma but may also be associated with oral cancers.

Local Manifestations of Systemic Disease

The mouth may show manifestations of systemic disorders such as the diffuse lip swelling, cobblestone buccal mucosa ulceration and glossitis found in Crohn's disease, or the glossitis and angular cheilitis seen in iron deficiency. Endogenous pigmentation may be found in Addison's disease or as circumoral pigmentation in Peutz–Jegher's syndrome. Oral ulceration and mucosal bleeding may be a manifestation of leukaemias, agranulocytosis or severe glandular fever.

GENERAL

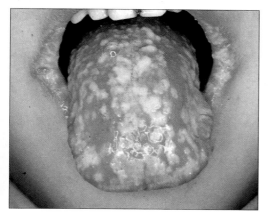

10.1   Oral thrush (*Candida albicans*). The most common sites for this infection in denture wearers are in the palate under the denture, and at the angles of the mouth as angular cheilitis. In debilitated and immunosuppressed patients and those on long-term broad spectrum antibiotics, oral and vaginal candidiasis may be difficult to control. The infection may affect the tongue, palate and oropharynx as a thick white 'curd-like' plaque which can be wiped off to leave a local area of erythema on the mucosa. Yeast hyphae are seen microscopically and antifungal agents such as nystatin are used locally with effect, provided the underlying cause is treated.

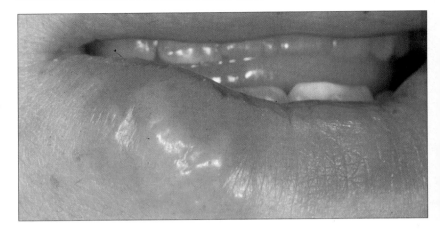

10.2 Cold sore (*Herpes simplex*). Primary infection with herpes type I virus often affects the oral mucous membrane and lips of young children and adults as a primary herpetic gingivo-stomatitis. A number of patients who have had the primary infection will develop recurrent infection, usually on the lips, with no systemic illness. There is usually a prodromal stage of several days, described as a 'tingling' on the lip margin, and topical application of acyclovir at this stage may avoid vesicular eruption. *Herpes* labialis may also be found in debilitated patients, after major surgery or when there is concomitant chronic illness or malignancy.

LIPS AND PALATE

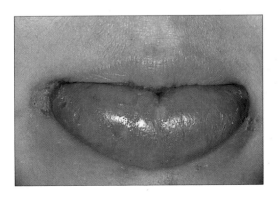

10.3 Macrocheilia. Oral manifestations of Crohn's disease include macrocheilia presenting as a diffuse, firm swelling of either the upper or lower lip. Surgery is contraindicated. Treatment of the disease may help the lip swelling.

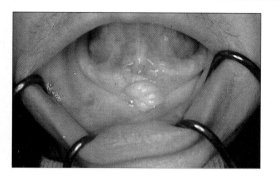

10.4 Squamous cell papilloma. This is a very common benign tumour of the oral mucosa. It is usually a solitary lesion, may vary in size and be sessile or pedunculated. It is not considered to be premalignant.

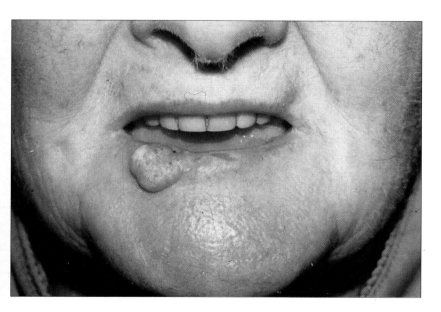

10.5 Carcinoma of the lip. These lesions most commonly present on the vermilion border of the lower lip. Their incidence has declined in the UK but is increasing among Caucasians in tropical climates. Some lip carcinomas are exophytic, others will ulcerate, but they are slow to metastasise to the submental and submandibular nodes. A **differential diagnosis** may include papilliferous wart, kerato–acanthoma, haemangioma, lymphangioma, *herpes* labialis or syphilitic chancre.

CLEFT LIP AND PALATE

This is one of the most common developmental abnormalities of the head and neck, with an incidence of 1 in 700 live births. The defects may be unilateral or bilateral, presenting as cleft lip with or without cleft palate, and cleft palate alone. Nasal regurgitation during neonatal feeding can usually be overcome with the use of special teats.

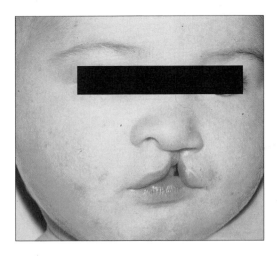

10.6   Cleft lip. A unilateral cleft lip (as shown) is repaired when the child is between 3 and 6 months old.

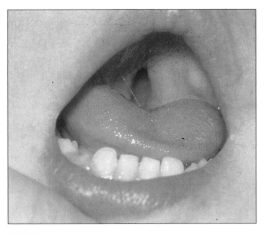

10.7   Cleft palate. Palatal defect closure is usually delayed until 18 months of age in order to ensure that speech will develop as normally as possible. To improve phonation and deglutination, further corrective operations may be required.

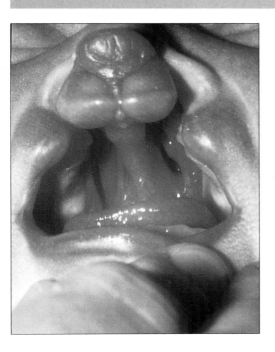

10.8 Bilateral cleft lip and palate. This is the most extreme form of this defect and requires major reconstructive surgery.

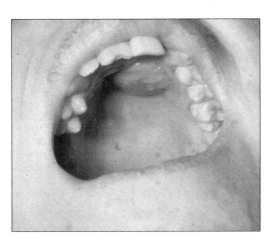

10.9 Apical abscess from lateral incisor tooth. The apex of this tooth is adjacent to the anterior hard palate and infection from the tooth or the retained root (as seen in this patient) will produce an abscess on the anterior hard palate, or pus may track under the periosteum to produce a swelling between hard and soft palate.

ORAL CAVITY

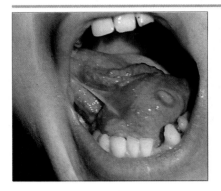

10.10 Ranula. This is a large mucus retention cyst found in the floor of the mouth. It will displace the tongue as it enlarges, producing a minor change in speech. It will transilluminate and should be widely decompressed into the floor of the mouth. It cannot be excised as it has no cyst lining.

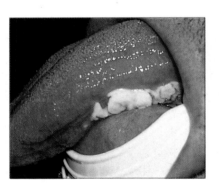

10.11 Leukoplakia. This is a white patch found in the mouth, with no known cause. It cannot be removed by rubbing. There is some pathological evidence to suggest that tobacco products, alcohol, Epstein–Barr or papilloma viruses may be associated with idiopathic leukoplakias. Malignant change is said to be found in 4% of leukoplakias, so regular review and biopsy of suspicious sites is required.

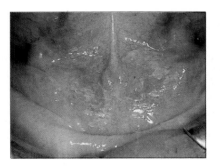

10.12 Erythroplakia. This is seen as a bright red, velvety plaque with an irregular outline on the oral mucosa, with no obvious cause. It may be intermingled with areas of leukoplakia as a leuko–erythroplakia. Histologically, it may contain areas of dysplasia, carcinoma *in situ* or early invasive carcinoma, so it must be regarded as highly premalignant, and excised.

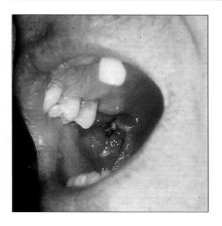

10.13 Carcinoma of the buccal mucosa. Tumours of the buccal mucosa are more common in the Indian subcontinent, and tend to occur in close relation to the site where a betel quid is lodged in the mouth. Chewing of betel is less common in the UK, where lesions may present as prolific or ulcerated masses.

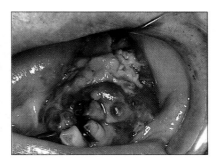

10.14 Carcinoma of the floor of mouth. Tumours often present in the anterior floor of mouth as indurated ulcers. This is a common site and the tumour may extend on to the tongue or into the alveolus. Abundant lymphatic drainage may produce early lymphatic spread.

TONGUE

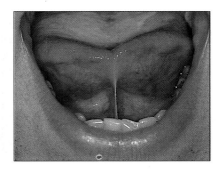

10.15 Tied tongue. In this condition the tongue is tethered to the floor of the mouth by a shortened frenulum. The patient cannot extend the tip of the tongue beyond the front teeth. Parents are often concerned that this abnormality will delay speech development but this is not the case in practice. It causes no symptoms but, for the sake of appearance, it is easy to cut the frenulum and thus mobilise the tongue.

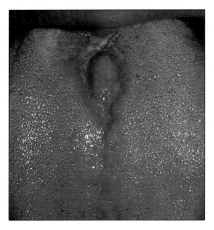

10.16 Median rhomboid glossitis. This asymptomatic lesion is located in the midline on the dorsum of the tongue, anterior to the foramen caecum. It has a characteristic diamond shape which is devoid of papillae, so it appears as a red, smooth or nodular mass. It used to be regarded as a developmental anomaly from the tuberculum impar, but current work suggests it is a localised chronic candidiasis which may respond to antifungal therapy.

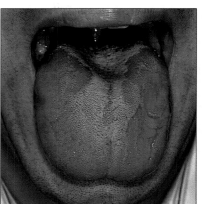

10.17 Geographic tongue. Large or small areas on the dorsal surface show atrophy of the filiform papillae, resulting in a smooth, red mucosal surface in which the fungiform papillae become visible as little red elevations. In a matter of weeks or months the area becomes normal again, but the lesion becomes apparent somewhere else on the tongue. Treatment is by simple reassurance that it is benign and does not require intervention.

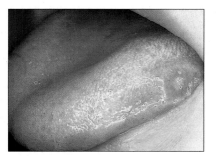

10.18 Aphthous ulcer of the tongue. This begins as a thickening on the side of the tongue, which breaks down after about 24 hours to form a small, punched-out ulcer, the raised rampart-like margins of which are associated with extreme pain. In the differential diagnosis, one must consider *Herpes zoster*, trauma, syphilis and tuberculosis.

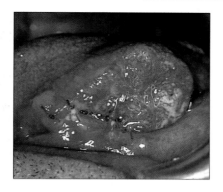

10.19 Carcinoma of the tongue.
This is a very common site for intra oral tumours. Carcinoma may present as a painless mass which may be deeply infiltrating, or as a painful, indurated ulcer with raised, rolled edges. The most common site is the lateral border of the tongue, and the anterior two thirds is more common than the posterior third. The abundance of lymphatics in the tongue influences the frequency and early spread to both ipsilateral and contralateral cervical lymph nodes.

GUMS AND JAW

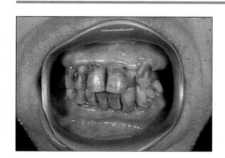

10.20 Gross dental caries and periodontal disease. This patient with a neglected dentition requires careful assessment prior to anaesthesia because of the risk of tooth fracture or tooth displacement during intubation, with a risk of inhalation of debris.

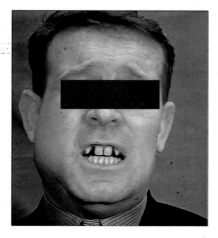

10.21 Oro-facial infections. Dental sepsis from a root apex, infection around an erupting wisdom tooth (pericoronitis) or an infected facial fracture may drain intra orally or track along tissue planes between muscle bellies or muscle and bone in the face and neck. This patient has associated **trismus** (inability to open the mouth due to tonic contracture of the muscles of the jaw). Severe deep-seated infections may result in pyrexia, pain, swelling, dysphagia and marked trismus. The airway may become embarrassed in severe cases of Ludwig's angina, when there is swelling of all tissues in the floor of the mouth with posterior displacement of the tongue.

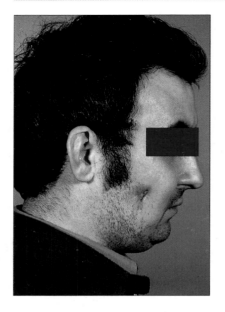

10.22 Facial sinus. A dental infection may progress into the soft tissues of the face, chin or neck and discharge through the overlying skin. The infection may appear to settle, but a persistently discharging sinus may be evident on the face (as seen in this patient). The sinus should not be excised; the original cause of the infection should be confirmed and treated, the sinus will then heal as a puckered scar which, if unsightly, may be improved at a later date.

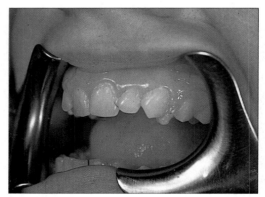

10.23 Epulis. This is a common soft tissue swelling of the gums. Common forms include **fibrous** (as shown), which is found as a sessile or pedunculated mass arising from the attached mucosa. A **vascular** epulis presents as a soft, red or purple fleshy swelling and is found most frequently during pregnancy. It resolves after parturition. **Giant cell** epulides are found at the extremes of life, usually on the anterior alveolar mucosa.

JAW CYSTS

Differential Diagnosis

- **Dentigerous cyst.** This cyst arises from the amelo–cemental junction of an unerupted tooth and is developed from the tooth follicle. It is most frequently found associated with an unerupted wisdom tooth. The swelling is slow growing and symptom-free unless it becomes infected.
- **Eruption cyst.** This is a bluish dentigerous cyst seen in the mouth lying over an erupting permanent tooth.
- **Keratocyst.** This is an uncommon cyst which is thought to arise from remnants of the dental lamina. It is usually symptom-free and enlarges into the marrow space without causing significant bony expansion.
- **Ameloblastoma.** This is a rare, locally invasive, tumour derived from odontogenic epithelium and is found most commonly in the mandibular molar region. It is slow growing, usually occurs in early adulthood, and causes bony expansion. Radiologically it appears as a multilocular radiolucency.

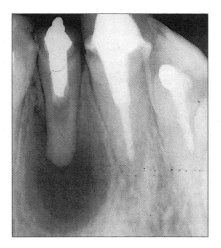 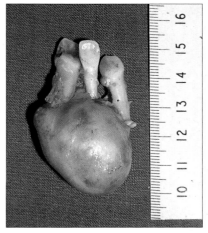

10.24 Dental cyst. This cyst is related to the root of a non-vital standing tooth (***left***) and represents about 60% of all jaw cysts. If the tooth is removed it may remain as a residual cyst and become infected. The pathological specimen shows removal of the cyst and associated teeth (***right***).

MALIGNANT TUMOURS

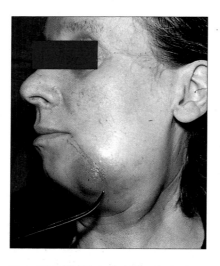

10.25 Osteogenic sarcoma. This is the most common primary malignant tumour of bone, but it is very rare in the jaw bones. The tumour usually presents in patients under 30 years of age, but may present in older patients as a complication of Paget's disease (as shown in this patient in whom there is secondary infection) or following radiotherapy. Radical surgery and extensive reconstruction may be required.

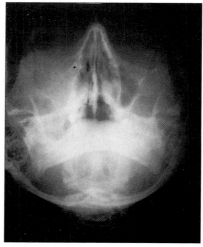

10.26 Carcinoma of the maxillary antrum. Antral tumours are uncommon and probably arise from the antral mucosa with an insidious onset and late presentation. The age of presentation may lie between 40 and 70 years, with an equal sex distribution. A radiograph shows an antral opacity and erosion of the antral walls. Presentation of this carcinoma depends on the direction of tumour growth. If **medial extension** occurs there may be blockage of the antral osteum with recurrent sinusitis or nasal obstruction and unilateral intermittent epistaxis or discharge. **Lateral extension** may present as a swelling of the face, which may have an inflamed appearance. **Superior extension** into the orbit causes proptosis, diplopia and epiphora, while **inferior extension** may mimic a local infective or cystic dental problem.

11.

SALIVARY GLANDS

There are **three principal pairs** of salivary glands (the **parotid**, the **submandibular** and the **sublingual**), in addition to multiple small, un-named glands scattered throughout the mucosa of the mouth, cheeks, lips and palate. Inflammatory conditions and tumours generally involve a single gland, although the principal exceptions to this are viral parotitis (mumps) and auto-immune diseases.

The **parotid gland** is enclosed in a sheath of deep cervical fascia which makes palpation difficult and means that any acute swelling is extremely painful. The parotid duct runs over the edge of the masseter muscle and enters the buccal mucosa opposite the second upper molar tooth. The facial nerve has an intimate relationship with the superficial part of the gland after leaving the stylomastoid foramen, and divides into its five constituent branches which emerge to supply the muscles of facial expression. The **differential diagnosis** of parotid lesions includes enlargement of the upper cervical lymph nodes and enlargement of the jugulo–digastric lymph node.

The **submandibular gland** has a superficial portion which fills most of the digastric triangle and extends upwards beneath the body of the mandible. The submandibular duct runs forwards to open in the floor of the mouth at the side of the frenulum of the tongue. The facial artery and vein and the cervical branch of the facial nerve run over the lateral border of the gland and the lingual and hypoglossal nerves lie deep to it. The submandibular gland secretes a mixture of both serous and mucous saliva.

The **sublingual gland**, smallest and least affected by disease, lies in the floor of the mouth adjacent to the submandibular duct into which it secretes.

Parotid Gland Anatomy

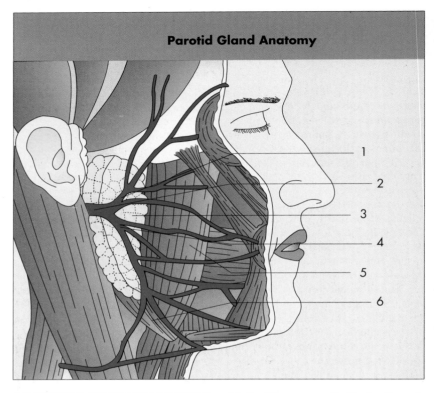

1 Temporofacial division
2 Facial nerve trunk
3 Deep lobe of parotid gland
4 Cervicofacial division
5 Masseter muscle
6 Posterior belly of digastric muscle

11.1 Diagrammatic illustration of parotid anatomy. The parotid gland is bounded by the zygomatic arch above, below by the angle of the mandible, posteriorly to it, is the anterior border of the sternocleidomastoid and anteriorly it extends over the masseter muscle.

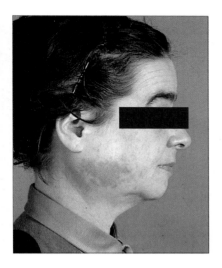

11.2 Acute parotitis. This elderly patient has a unilateral swelling in the region of the parotid gland which is exquisitely tender. The overlying skin is stretched, shiny and reddened, and trismus is marked. The inflamed and patulous parotid duct orifice may evoke a gush of pus when the gland is gently milked. The organism usually responsible is *Staphylococcus*. Rarely, a parotid abscess can develop, but fluctuation is a late sign because of the tight overlying fascia. This condition is uncommon now but the postoperative, elderly, debilitated and dehydrated patient is susceptible. Treatment is directed at frequent mouth washes, coating the gums with a viscous antiseptic such as bromo-glycerol and promotion of salivation by sialogogues.

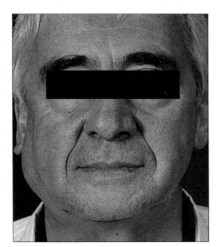
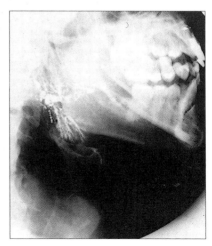

11.3 Sialectasis. This patient presented with intermittent episodes of pain and distension of the parotid gland due to stasis and infection (**left**). The sialogram (**right**) is diagnostic and shows a dilated and distended duct system. An autoimmune basis for swelling of the parotid gland must be excluded. The patient was treated expectantly but, if severely symptomatic, superficial parotidectomy may be required.

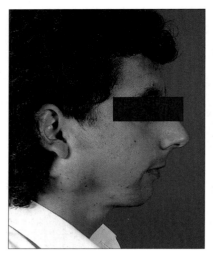

11.4 Pleomorphic adenoma. This usually affects the superficial portion of the parotid gland and is found most frequently in middle-aged adults. These tumours are slow growing and may reach a substantial size without causing symptoms. They are not frankly malignant and do not invade or metastasise. However, there is a high incidence of recurrence if the lesion is incompletely excised. This patient presented with a firm swelling in the lower part of the parotid gland. Other diagnoses such as a simple dermoid, sebaceous cyst or cervical lymph node should be considered. Superficial parotidectomy was carried out with no evidence of recurrence five years after surgery.

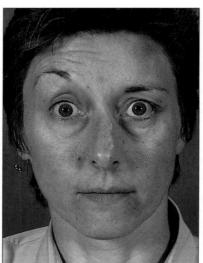
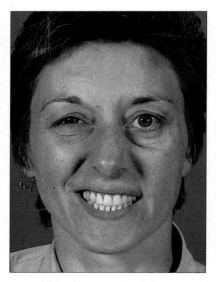

11.5 Facial nerve palsy. This patient has a partial facial nerve palsy following parotid surgery which required secondary corrective treatment. Damage to the nerve can be avoided per-operatively by its accurate identification using electro-stimulation. Facial palsy can also be due to invasion of the facial nerve, which is uncommon but diagnostic of malignancy.

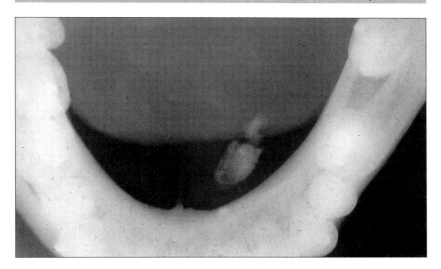

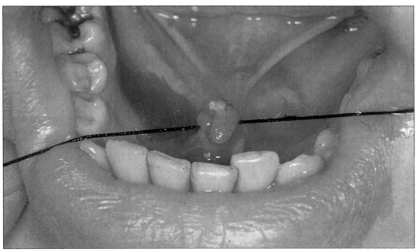

11.6 Submandibular gland sialolithiasis. This patient had a recurrent swelling in the submandibular area at meal times which appeared rapidly and slowly subsided. This was caused by subtotal obstruction of the duct by a calculus which could be felt by bimanual palpation and seen on a radiograph of the floor of the mouth (**top**). This was dealt with by opening the duct and extracting the calculus (**bottom**).

12.

PHARYNX

The pharynx is divided into the **nasopharynx**, which extends from the base of the skull to the soft palate and contains lymphoid tissue on the posterior wall (adenoids), the **oropharynx**, which opens anteriorly into the mouth and extends from the soft palate to the tip of the epiglottis, and the **hypopharynx**, which is bounded above by the tip of the epiglottis and extends to the level of the cricoid cartilage.

The most common conditions affecting the **nasopharynx** are **adenoid hypertrophy** and **neoplasia**. Presenting features may include blockage of the Eustachian tube, bleeding from tumours, or enlargement of the cervical lymph nodes.

Oropharyngeal lesions have to be large before they obstruct swallowing and, unlike those in the mouth, they frequently cause pain.

Hypopharyngeal pathology usually presents with a sensation of 'something being there'.

Diagnosis
Methods of diagnosis include:
- Indirect pharyngoscopy.
- Plain lateral radiography.
- Barium swallow.

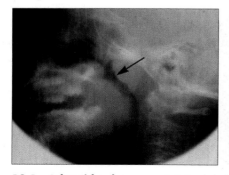 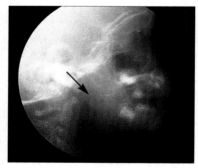

12.1 Adenoid enlargement. Lateral skull radiography in this child demonstrates enlargement of the adenoids which were simply curetted (**left**). Occlusion of the nasopharyngeal space is not uncommon (**right**). The most common complication of adenoidectomy is postoperative haemorrhage.

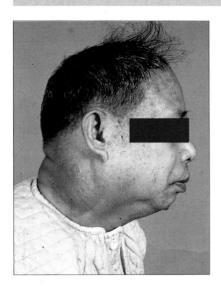

12.2   Nasopharyngeal carcinoma.
This is one of the most common carcinomas in South-East Asia, particularly in populations of Chinese extraction. It is a squamous cell carcinoma which may present late with erosion of the base of the skull or with cervical lymph node metastases as shown in this patient.

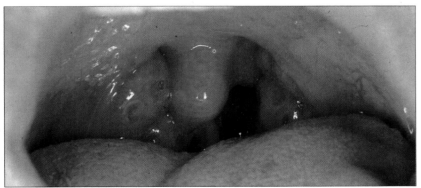

12.3   Acute tonsillitis. Bacterial tonsillitis due to *beta-haemolytic Streptococci* is a condition of childhood and adolescence. The tonsils pictured here are inflamed and enlarged with muco-pus in the crypts. The patient was treated with analgesia and oral penicillin for 5 days. The **differential diagnosis** includes acute viral pharyngitis and infectious mononucleosis. Failure of tonsillitis to settle on appropriate antimicrobial therapy may result in the development of a peri-tonsillar abscess and possible airway obstruction (quinsy). Parenteral penicillin may be effective in the early stages of abscess formation but the abscess may have to be dealt with by stab incision under local anaesthesia or by tonsillectomy under general anaesthesia.

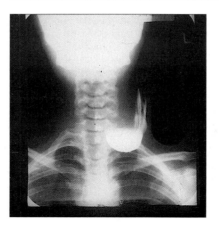

12.4 Pharyngeal pouch. The barium swallow shows a fluid level in the pharyngeal pouch which is caused by mucosal herniation through the lower pharyngeal muscles (Killian's dehiscence), which gradually enlarges with retained food. The underlying pathophysiology, usually affecting the elderly, is lack of coordination between contraction of the pharynx and relaxation of the upper oesophageal sphincter. The pouch is dissected following exploration of the neck. Treatment consists of excision of the pouch, repair of the defect and division of the crico–pharyngeal muscle (myotomy).

Section 4

Thorax

13.

LUNGS AND CHEST WALL

PNEUMONIA

In surgical practice, infection of the lung may mimic the signs of intra-abdominal pathology and can arise as a complication of anaesthesia or surgery. Following aspiration of fluid, food or secretions, there is collapse of the basal segments of the right lower lobe (**aspiration pneumonia**). These same segments are often affected in the post-operative period by **atelectasis,** in which collapse of the alveolar spaces occurs beyond obstructed bronchioles. If the early signs of this condition are not recognised (postoperative pyrexia, dullness to percussion, diminished breath sounds, bronchial breathing and fine crepitations at the affected base), they may progress and evolve into **lobar pneumonia.**

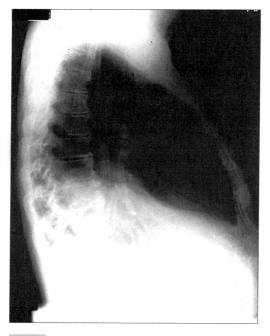

13.1   Lobar pneumonia.
A lateral chest radiograph showing opacification of the right base. The main pathogen isolated on bacterial culture was *Streptococcus pneumoniae*. This responded to physiotherapy and antibiotic treatment with ampicillin.

Acute respiratory distress may result from:
- Pulmonary embolus.
- Pulmonary oedema (acute left ventricular failure).
- Fat embolus.
- Adult respiratory distress syndrome (ARDS).

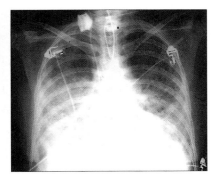

13.2 ARDS. Chest radiograph of a patient who developed acute respiratory failure 5 days after admission to hospital having sustained a fractured right femur. This patient required prolonged ventilatory support following fixation of the fracture. Note the fluffy opacification in both lung fields, the presence of a tracheostomy tube, a central venous line and a nasogastric tube.

PLEURA

Pneumothorax may develop when air leaks from the lung, enters through the injured chest wall or enters through a perforated oesophagus. **Spontaneous pneumothorax** is the most common form, but if small, this may not require active treatment. If the pneumothorax is large or is under tension, it will require treatment by insertion of an intercostal drain. A **tension pneumothorax** which causes mediastinal shift or venous obstruction may require the urgent insertion of a large-bore needle before formal drainage is instituted. **Recurrent spontaneous pneumothorax** will require a definitive procedure such as pleurectomy, or pleurodesis which involves the instillation of an irritant substance into the pleural cavity.

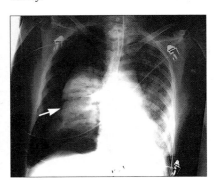

13.3 Spontaneous pneumothorax. Chest radiograph showing collapse of the right lung. The patient presented with pain and dyspnoea, and examination revealed a hyper-resonant right chest and reduced breath sounds on auscultation. The lung reinflated completely following insertion of a chest drain connected to an underwater seal.

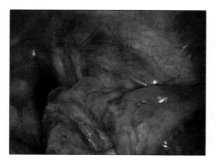 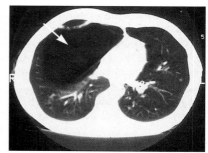

13.4 Bulla of the lung. This thoracoscopic examination (*left*) in a 45-year-old man demonstrates a bulla on the pleural surface of the right lung. Such lesions are found with increasing age and, as the CT scan demonstrates (*right*), may reach a substantial size by the time they become symptomatic. These should not be mistaken for a pneumothorax, since insertion of a chest drain would be inappropriate.

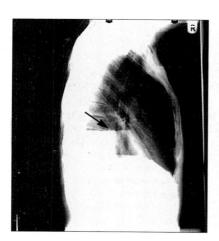 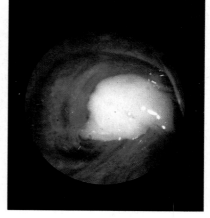

13.5 Empyema. This lateral chest radiograph (*left*) shows an air fluid level in the right chest. The patient was coughing up copious amounts of sputum and the accompanying bronchoscopy (*right*) shows pus in the right main bronchus from a bronchopleural fistula. The most common cause of pus in the pleural cavity is an underlying **pneumonia**. Infection can also be introduced from a **lung abscess** or from outside the chest as a result of a **penetrating injury**. Infection may also spread from the mediastinum or from a **subphrenic abscess**.

LUNG TUMOURS

The benign lung tumours, adenoma, carcinoid, hamartoma and haemangioma, are uncommonly found. **Primary lung cancer** is the most common cause of death from malignancy in both sexes.

Secondary tumours of the lung are very common, and may be the first presentation of a primary tumour. Frequent primary sites include breast, colon, bone (sarcoma) and skin (melanoma).

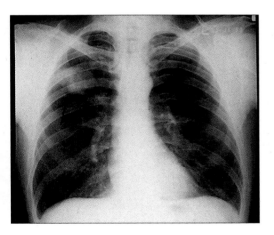

13.6 Primary lung carcinoma. Chest radiograph showing an opacity in the periphery of the right upper lobe. This patient presented with haemoptysis. Although the tumour was not visible at bronchoscopy, brushings taken from the segmental bronchus confirmed the presence of a well-differentiated adenocarcinoma.

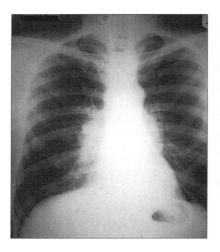
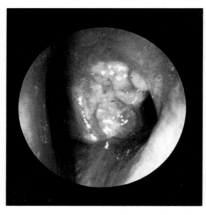

13.7 Bronchial carcinoma. Chest radiograph (***left***) demonstrating the presence of a right hilar mass. Bronchoscopy (***right)*** in this patient, who presented with haemoptysis, increasing dyspnoea and weight loss, demonstrates a bronchial carcinoma involving the carina.

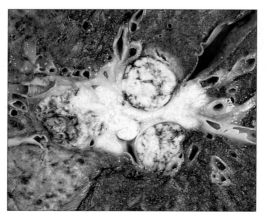

13.8 Bronchial carcinoma. This patient presented with a recurrent cough and hoarseness which was shown to be due to vocal cord paralysis from left recurrent laryngeal nerve involvement. The diagnosis of bronchial carcinoma was made in life at bronchoscopy. The postmortem specimen shows a locally infiltrative tumour associated with involvement of the adjacent lymph nodes.

TRAUMA

The chest wall is commonly involved in trauma, and injuries can be classified as **penetrating** or **blunt**. Injuries range from simple rib fractures from a direct blow to **flail chest**, in which a crushing injury to the rib cage has resulted in multiple rib fractures.

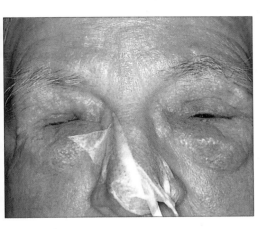

13.9 Surgical emphysema. This patient sustained a direct blow to the left side of the chest during an assault and examination revealed some soft tissue swelling and crepitus on palpation of the head, neck and periorbital region. The associated chest radiograph showed no obvious pneumothorax but there were areas of lucency in the soft tissues characteristic of surgical emphysema.

14.

HEART AND GREAT VESSELS

CONGENITAL HEART DISEASE

Congenital heart disease occurs in about 6 to 8 per 1000 live births and is classified into **cyanotic** and **non-cyanotic**. The presence of cyanotic heart disease (large right-to-left shunts) usually indicates the need for urgent surgical intervention to improve systemic oxygenation. Although symptoms may not become apparent until late in life, the abnormality usually presents in childhood, and severe malformations in the neonatal period also have the highest attendant surgical mortality.

Cardinal symptoms and signs include: cyanosis, dyspnoea/tachypnoea, tachycardia, hypotension, peripheral oedema, failure to thrive, poor exercise tolerance and syncope. The child may exhibit a typical crouching position, lateral displacement of the cardiac apex, ventricular heaves, cardiac murmurs and thrills, respiratory crepitations and pitting oedema.

Diagnosis
- General examination.
- Clinical examination of the heart and lungs.
- Electrocardiography.
- Chest radiography.
- Echocardiography with Doppler flow imaging.
- Cardiac catheterisation and cineangiography.

The **ductus arteriosus** allows pulmonary artery blood to bypass the airless lungs during intra-uterine life. Failure of normal closure results in left-to-right shunting of systemic blood into the pulmonary circulation, as pulmonary vascular resistance falls after birth. This may produce cardiac failure in infancy, requiring urgent surgery. More commonly, the shunt is well tolerated and the characteristic 'machinery' murmur in the second left interspace is the reason for referral. Surgery carries little risk and is always advised.

Atrial septal defect is probably the most frequent single congenital malformation of the heart encountered in clinical practice; it is more common in girls. **Salient features** include increased pulmonary blood flow, a delayed pulmonary second sound and radiological evidence of pulmonary plaeonaemia. The defect is of two types: **ostium primum** in which the defect is low down in the septum, the base being formed by the mitral and tricuspid valves which may also be malformed; and **ostium secundum,** in which the defect is higher so that only the septum is involved.

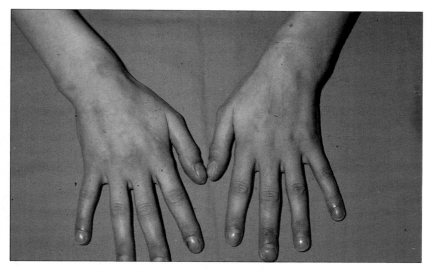

14.1 Cyanotic heart disease. This patient's hands demonstrate gross cyanosis and clubbing. The congenital heart disease was due to a ventricular septal defect (VSD). These defects cause a left-to-right shunt because left ventricular pressure is higher than right ventricular pressure during systole, giving rise to a loud pan-systolic murmur, audible in the left fourth intercostal space, associated with a thrill. Excessive pulmonary blood flow results in pulmonary hypertension, eventual cessation and then reversal of the shunting through the VSD **(Eisenmenger syndrome).** This causes cyanosis and is inoperable, requiring combined heart and lung transplantation.

Fallot's Tetralogy

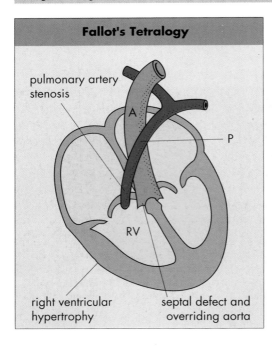

pulmonary artery stenosis

A

P

RV

right ventricular hypertrophy

septal defect and overriding aorta

14.2 Fallot's tetralogy. The diagrammatic illustration shows (a) normal equal division of the truncus arteriosus into the aorta (A) and pulmonary artery (P); and in (b) Fallot's tetralogy, where the dividing septum is off-centre, causing the aorta to be larger than normal and to override the right ventricle (RV). The pulmonary artery is smaller than normal. Since the truncus septum is not central, it fails to meet the intra-ventricular septum, thus leaving a ventricular septal defect.

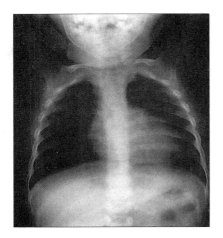

14.3 Fallot's tetralogy. The chest radiograph shows reduced lung field vascularity, a shallow main pulmonary segment and a right-sided aortic knuckle. Both ventricles are at systemic pressure and the right ventricle is hypertrophic. Right-to-left shunting of blood across the VSD results in cyanosis. Palliative shunting between the systemic and pulmonary circulation (Blalock–Taussig shunt) may be undertaken in the first two years of life for severe cyanosis since there is a risk of spontaneous intravascular thrombosis from polycythaemia. Total correction is usually advised before the child reaches school age. Operative mortality is approximately 5%.

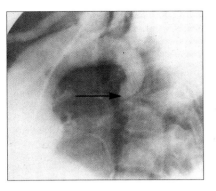 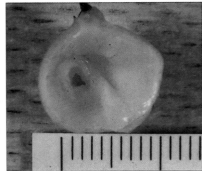

14.4 Coarctation of the aorta. This arch aortogram (**left**) shows the typical narrowing of the aorta, which usually occurs just beyond the origin of the left subclavian artery. The diagnosis is suggested by absent or delayed femoral pulses. In older patients, rib notching is often seen on radiological examination. About 50% of patients die within the first year of life from cardiac failure, and complications from proximal hypertension frequently lead to death in early adult life. Operation is always advised and is undertaken through a left lateral thoracotomy. The aorta is temporarily cross-clamped above and below the narrowed segment, which is resected and the aortic ends sutured primarily. The resected specimen of the aorta is shown (**right**).

AORTIC AND MITRAL VALVE DISEASE

Depending on the aetiology and the valve affected, stenosis, regurgitation or both may occur, and will determine the clinical findings.

Causes of Valvular Disease
Congenital
Acquired
- Rheumatic fever.
- Pancarditis.
- Infective endocarditis.
- Chordal rupture.
- Leaflet degeneration.
- Infarction or rupture of papillary muscle.
- Left ventricular dilatation in severe cardiac failure.
- Dissecting thoracic aortic aneurysm.

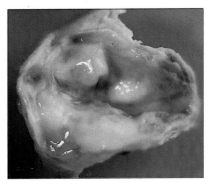

14.5   Aortic stenosis. This pathological specimen shows destruction of a bicuspid aortic valve resulting in severe stenosis. Clinically the patient suffered from syncopal attacks and exercise-induced angina. A systolic ejection type murmur was audible in the second right interspace, transmitted into the neck. Radiography may show calcification of the valve and an enlarged left ventricle.

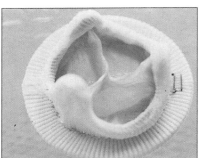

14.6   Aortic valve. There are many types of prosthetic valves available, but the one shown is a bio-prosthetic porcine valve which replaces the stenosed valve in the aortic annulus. The patient requires long-term warfarinisation to maintain valve function and prevent recurrent embolic episodes.

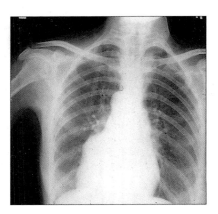

14.7   Mitral valve stenosis. Chest radiograph shows typical prominence of the left atrium and pulmonary congestion. Rheumatic fever has been responsible for the development of the abnormality in this patient, who presented with atrial fibrillation. Doppler imaging and echocardiography are extremely useful in determining the extent of valvular disease.

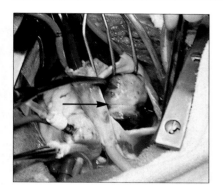

14.8 Atrial myxoma. This condition is a rare presentation of atrial fibrillation and embolic disease. The diagnosis is established by echocardiography. The operative photograph shows a left atrial myxoma (arrow) with the patient on cardiopulmonary bypass, and the left atrium opened.

ISCHAEMIC HEART DISEASE

Surgery for coronary artery disease has become extremely common in most Western countries. **Angina pectoris** is the usual indication for surgery, and most surgeons now agree that surgery should be offered where symptoms persist or interfere with activities in spite of adequate medical therapy. It is now widely accepted that triple vessel disease and left main coronary artery disease, particularly when associated with impaired left ventricular function, have a better long-term prognosis with surgical treatment and long-term aspirin than with medical therapy alone.

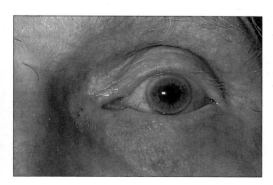

14.9 Arcus senilis. This 66-year-old male has had three myocardial infarctions precipitated by hyperlipidaemia and coronary artery disease. This eye sign is a common finding in this condition and may be associated with cutaneous xantholasma.

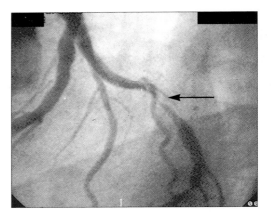

14.10 Coronary artery stenosis. In a 61-year-old patient with unstable angina and dyspnoea on minimal exercise, coronary angiography – the mainstay of diagnosis – shows an isolated stenosis of the circumflex artery (arrow). This can be managed by coronary angioplasty, placement of a stent or by coronary artery bypass grafting (CABG).

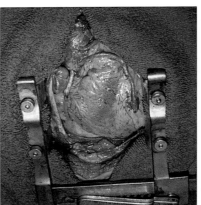

14.11 Multivessel disease. This operative photograph shows the three main coronary vessels to have been bypass grafted with saphenous vein. Alternatively, the internal mammary artery can be used to restore an adequate flow to the vessels.

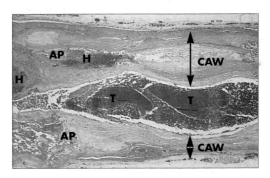

14.12 Coronary artery stenosis. Failure to bypass stenotic coronary artery segments may result in sudden occlusion by plaque thrombosis (shown in this pathological specimen) causing myocardial infarction or death. CAW = coronary artery wall; AP = atheromatous plaque; H = haemorrhage into atheromatous plaque; T = coronary artery thrombosis caused by sudden haemorrhage into atheromatous plaque.

HYPERTENSION

In Western civilisation the normal blood pressure gradually rises with age, and hypertension is present in about 15 per cent of the population. In approximately 80–90 per cent of patients with hypertension, even the use of refined diagnostic methods will not establish an underlying aetiology (**primary hypertension**). Its basis is multifactorial and may be related to inheritance, geography, and salt intake.

In the remaining 10–20 per cent of patients, a rational approach to finding an underlying aetiology for **secondary hypertension** is important because cure is often possible; the search is most likely to be rewarded in children and young adults.

Differential Diagnosis of Hypertension
- Coarctation of the aorta.
- Aortic dissection.
- Renal disease (parenchymous, polycystic or renal artery stenosis) (*Section 8: Urology*).
- Endocrine (oral contraception, oestrogen therapy, phaeochromocytoma, Cushing's syndrome, Conn's syndrome) (*Section 7: Endocrinology*).
- Pregnancy.

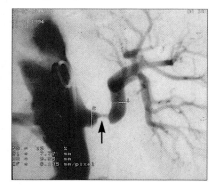 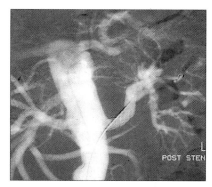

14.13   Renal artery stenosis. Renal artery stenosis is an uncommon but important and treatable cause of hypertension and/or renal failure. Untreated stenosis may progress to occlusion (which is untreatable). Renal artery stenosis arises from either **atherosclerosis** or **fibromuscular dysplasia**. The former is part of generalised atheromatous disease and is really an extension of aortic disease found in the elderly. The lesions are typically ostial, very hard and therefore not amenable to percutaneous techniques. Surgical bypass is required. By contrast, fibromuscular dysplasia is typically found in young women, occurs in the midpoint of the renal artery (**left**) and is amenable to PTA and stenting (**right**).

15.

MEDIASTINUM

The mediastinum is divided into four non-anatomical compartments: the superior, anterior, middle and posterior mediastinum. These titles are used for descriptive purposes only. Although mediastinal masses are often discovered as an incidental finding on chest radiography, suspicious symptoms may arise when a mass lesion causes pressure on adjacent structures such as the oesophagus, causing **dysphagia**; the trachea, causing **stridor**; the superior vena cava, causing **venous congestion** in the upper half of the body; or the recurrent laryngeal nerve, causing **hoarseness**.

Differential Diagnosis of Abnormal Mediastinal Shadowing on Chest Radiography

- Retrosternal thyroid.
- Aortic aneurysm.
- Aortic dissection.
- Thymic tumour or cyst.
- Lymphadenopathy.
- Pericardial effusion.
- Teratoma.
- Neurofibroma.
- Mediastinal abscess.
- Dermoid cyst.
- Mega-oesophagus associated with achalasia.

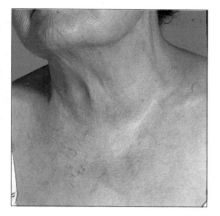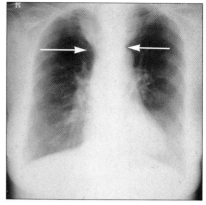

15.1 Retrosternal thyroid. A 42-year-old woman with no obvious goitre (*left*) has an upper mediastinal shadow on the chest radiograph (*right*). The thyroid is retrosternal because it lies below the level of the clavicles. Most retrosternal goitres can be removed through a transverse cervical incision, but occasionally a manubrial sternotomy is required to remove the gland.

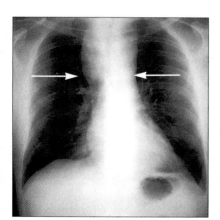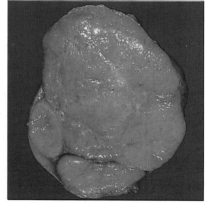

15.2 Thymoma. The chest radiograph in a 37-year-old male with myasthenia gravis shows a shadow in the anterior–superior space (*left*). The pathological specimen shows enlargement of both lobes of the thymus gland (*right*). Although thymomas are not exclusively associated with myasthenia gravis, this patient's neurological condition improved dramatically following gland removal through a median sternotomy.

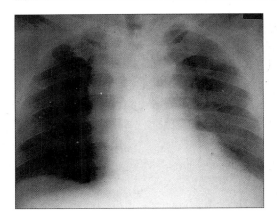

15.3 Traumatic aortic dissection. Immediate chest radiography in this motorcyclist involved in a road traffic accident demonstrated a grossly widened mediastinum. Aortography confirmed an aortic dissection and emergency thoracotomy necessitated prosthetic replacement. A high degree of suspicion is required to make the diagnosis bearing in mind the mechanism of injury.

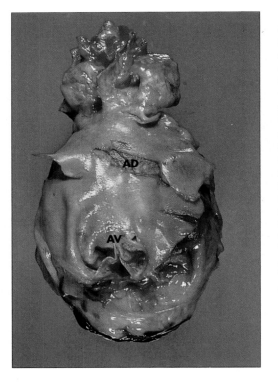

15.4 Dissecting aortic aneurysm. The chest radiograph showed a large aortic aneurysm in a patient complaining of dyspnoea. Chest auscultation revealed widespread crepitations and a pan-diastolic murmur associated with aortic regurgitation, which was secondary to dilatation of the aortic root. Before aortic arch reconstruction and aortic valve replacement could be undertaken, the aorta dissected causing severe, tearing back pain and from which the patient succumbed. The start of the aortic dissection (AD) is indicated. The aortic valve (AV) is also abnormal in that it is bicuspid.

16.

OESOPHAGUS

The **oesophagus** is a hollow muscular tube, 25 cm in length, which extends from the upper oesophageal sphincter of the cricopharyngous muscle (3–4 cm long) to the oesophago–gastric junction, the final 2–4 cm lying within the abdomen. It has **cervical**, **thoracic** and **abdominal** portions. Squamous epithelium lines the oesophageal mucosa except for the distal 1–2 cm, which is lined with columnar epithelium. There are two oesophageal **sphincters**, the lower of which is detected as a high-pressure zone on manometry, is atonically closed at rest, and is located in the region of the oesophageal hiatus and diaphragm.

The **principal symptoms** of **oesophageal disease** are:

- Dysphagia.
- Heartburn.
- Regurgitation.
- Retrosternal pain.
- Oesophageal spasm.

Differential Diagnosis of Dysphagia

Luminal
- Foreign body.

Intramural
- Atresia.
- Malignant stricture.
- Achalasia.
- Oesophageal web (Plummer–Vinson syndrome).
- Inflammatory stricture.
- Benign tumour.
- Pharyngeal pouch.

Extrinsic
- Retrosternal goitre.
- Aortic aneurysm.
- Paraoesophageal lymphadenopathy.
- Bronchial carcinoma.

General
- Myasthenia gravis.
- Bulbar poliomyelitis.
- Hysteria.
- Bulbar palsy.
- Diphtheria.

Diagnosis
- General examination.
- Chest radiograph.
- Upper gastrointestinal endoscopy, biopsy and epithelial brushings.
- Barium swallow.
- Manometry.
- pH studies.
- Computerised tomography.
- Laparoscopy.
- Bronchoscopy.
- Endoluminal ultrasound.

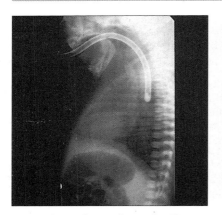 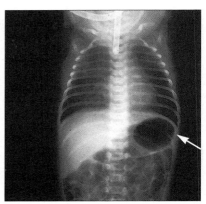

16.1 Oesophageal atresia. The most common congenital anomaly is atresia with an associated tracheo–oesophageal fistula. Atresia occurs in 1 in 2500 births and, in over half the cases, there is maternal hydramnios. A neonate usually presents with excess salivation, attacks of cyanosis and coughing. The diagnosis is confirmed by inability to pass a soft nasogastric tube more than 10 cm from the lips (***left***). The plain abdominal radiograph shows severe gaseous distension caused by a tracheo–oesophageal fistula (***right***). Following diagnosis, surgical repair is required urgently to prevent aspiration pneumonia.

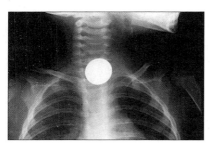

16.2 Swallowed foreign body. This child presented with painful dysphagia caused by the accidental ingestion of a coin. The principal complication is perforation of the mediastinum. It is important to view chest radiography in two planes, to place the foreign body in the oesophagus. The coin was removed under general anaesthesia and rigid oesophagoscopy.

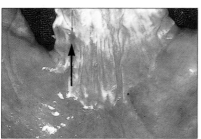

16.3 Mallory–Weiss tear. This pathological specimen of the oesophago–gastric junction shows a mucosal tear in the lateral position in a patient who presented with a small haematemesis, caused by several episodes of retching. This was managed expectantly with an H_2 receptor antagonist, but the patient, who was an arteriopath, succumbed from a myocardial infarction.

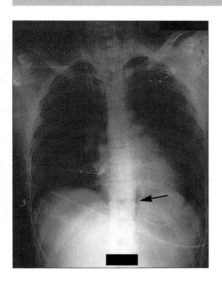

16.4 Oesophageal perforation.
The chest radiograph demonstrates pneumomediastinum (arrow) secondary to a perforated oesophagus. Following violent repeated vomiting after a large meal, the patient developed severe pain in the chest and the dorsal region of the spine. The patient subsequently collapsed and became cyanosed. Surgical emphysema was palpable in the left side of the neck. In this patient, oesophageal perforation was of a spontaneous nature (**Boerhaave's syndrome**), but other causes of perforation include swallowed foreign body; iatrogenic trauma from oesophagoscopic bouginage or biopsy, injection sclerotherapy; caustic oesophagitis and penetrating trauma.

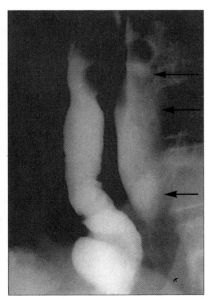

16.5 Oesophageal perforation. A
water soluble contrast study confirms the presence of perforation of the upper third of the oesophagus following a difficult endoscopy. Contrast is tracking posteriorly in the mediastinum (arrows).

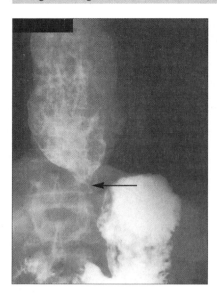

16.6 Achalasia. This barium swallow shows a dilated oesophagus ending in a chronically narrowed cardio–oesophageal junction (arrow), with food residue in the mega-oesophagus. The annual incidence of this condition is less than 1 per 100,000 population, and it is more common in women of middle age. Progressive dysphagia, particularly for fluids, causing regurgitation and recurrent aspiration pneumonia, are the main diagnostic indicators of the condition.

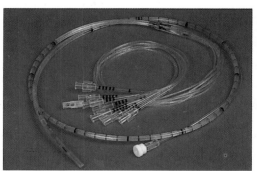

16.7 Oesophageal manometry. A multi-lumen tube is connected to a series of pressure transducers to determine the intra-luminal pressure at various levels in the oesophagus. The **aetiology of achalasia** is failure of neuromuscular relaxation at the lower oesophageal sphincter which, in turn, causes proximal dilatation, tortuosity, incoordination of peristalsis and hypertrophy of the oesophagus. A pressure of greater than **50 mmHg** in the lower oesophageal sphincter is **diagnostic of achalasia**. Treatment can be undertaken by forcible dilatation using hydrostatic, pneumatic or mechanical means. Cardiomyotomy (**Heller's operation**) is employed if dilatation fails, and can be carried out using an open or laparoscopic approach from the abdomen or the thorax.

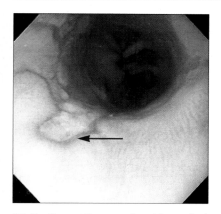

16.8 Barrett's oesophagitis and ulcer. In this condition, the lower oesophagus becomes lined with columnar epithelium as a metaplastic response to the chronic irritation. Endoscopically, it is often confused with hiatus hernia with which it may frequently co-exist (as shown), but it is easily recognised because of the tongues of gastric-type epithelium creeping up the oesophagus. Ulceration occurs at the squamo–columnar junction and may be complicated by bleeding, perforation or stricture formation. Biopsy is mandatory as the condition in premalignant, with 10% of patients developing an adenocarcinoma. Annual surveillance is required and treatment of ulceration (arrow) is by omeprazole.

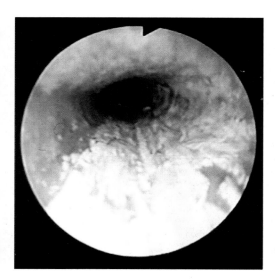

16.9 Oesophageal candidiasis. This is a florid example. It is often a sign of debilitating disease and is not infrequently associated with carcinoma of the stomach.

Classification of Oesophageal Neoplasms

Benign

- Leiomyoma.
- Fibroma.
- Neurofibroma.
- Lipoma.
- Haemangioma.

Malignant

- Carcinoma.
- Adenocarcinoma.
- Leiomyosarcoma.
- Secondary.

Oesophageal carcinoma has a variable incidence worldwide, but it is particularly common in South East Asia, Iran, Africa and the West Indies. **Predisposing factors** include: chronic irritation, alcohol, tobacco chewing, smoking, genetic factors, dietary factors (nitrosamines), aflatoxin, Plummer–Vinson syndrome, achalasia, hiatus hernia, Barrett's oesophagus and corrosive strictures. More than 90 per cent of oesophageal carcinomas are of the squamous type and predominate in the middle third of the oesophagus. Adenocarcinomas arise at the oesophago–gastric junction or in a Barrett's oesophagus.

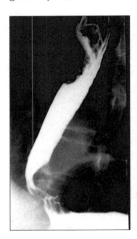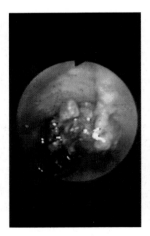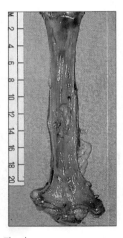

16.10 Squamous cell carcinoma of the oesophagus. This barium examination in a 48-year-old demonstrates a polypoidal lesion in the middle third of the oesophagus causing progressive dysphagia for solids (***left***). Biopsy and epithelial brushings at endoscopy confirmed the existence of a squamous cell carcinoma (***middle***). Following rigid bronchoscopy and laparoscopy which did not show evidence of either carinal involvement or peritoneal dissemination, this patient underwent oesophagectomy (***right***) and restoration of intestinal continuity by pulling up a mobilised stomach.

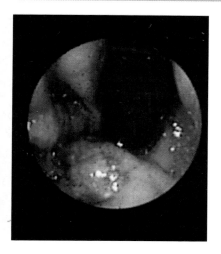

16.11 Adenocarcinoma of the oesophagus. This is the endoscopic appearance (with the endoscope retroflexed and viewing the cardia from the stomach) of an ulcerated polypoidal circumferential lesion in an elderly patient which caused haematemesis and progressive dysphagia for solids. Endoscopic biopsy confirmed an adenocarcinoma which required initial dilatation of the oesophagus to improve swallowing. Laparoscopy and laparoscopic ultrasonography demonstrated the presence of multiple hepatic metastases which precluded major thoraco–abdominal surgery. The patient was well palliated with laser therapy.

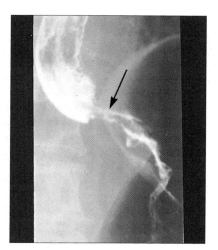

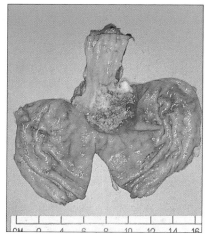

16.12 Adenocarcinoma of the oesophagus. A barium meal (*left*) performed for dysphagia shows a stricture (arrow) at the cardio–oesophageal junction which was confirmed as malignant by endoscopic brushings and biopsy. The resected specimen of oesophagus and stomach shows a tumour at the oesophago–gastric junction (*right*). Prognosis is poor, with a five-year survival expectation of 10%.

17.

DIAPHRAGMATIC HERNIAS

The diaphragm separating the thoracic and abdominal cavities allows the passage of three major structures: the **inferior vena cava** at the level of the eighth thoracic vertebra (T_8); the **oesophagus** (T_{10}); and the **aorta** (T_{12}).

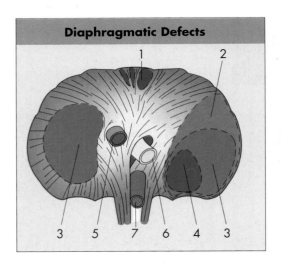

Diaphragmatic Defects

1 Morgagni defect
2 Hemi-diaphragmatic
   agenesis
3 Large Bochdalek
   defect
4 Bochdalek defect
5 Inferior vena cava (T_8)
6 Oesophagus (T_{10})
7 Aorta (T_{12})

17.1 Congenital diaphragmatic hernia.
Diagrammatic illustration shows the potential sites of herniation of the abdominal contents through the diaphragm, caused by embryological failure to fuse its component parts. Hernias may occur through the foramen of Morgagni (between the xiphoid and the costal origins); through the foramen of Bochdalek (a defect in the pleural–peritoneal canal); through a deficiency in the whole of the central tendon; and through a large oesophageal hiatus.

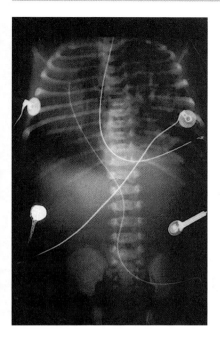

17.2 Congenital diaphragmatic hernia. The abnormality affects the left side in 85% of cases. It is now being diagnosed by antenatal ultrasound in many foetuses. Presentation in the neonatal period is usually with severe respiratory distress. Physical examination reveals a scaphoid abdomen. Air entry on the affected side is diminished and occasionally bowel sounds can be heard in the chest. Chest radiography is usually diagnostic, particularly if a nasogastric tube is seen entering the thoracic stomach. Mediastinal shift can result in serious cardiovascular instability. Treatment has now moved from immediate repair after birth to medical stabilisation for a number of days before closure of the diaphragmatic defect. Despite improvements in neonatal intensive care, including high frequency oscillation ventilation and extracorporeal oxygenation (ECMO), the mortality remains close to 50%.

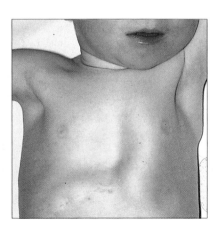

17.3 Chest deformity post-diaphragmatic hernia repair. This five-year-old boy had complete agenesis of his right hemi-diaphragm which was repaired with a dural patch. The repair has subsequently caused restriction in thoracic cage growth, leading to this deformity.

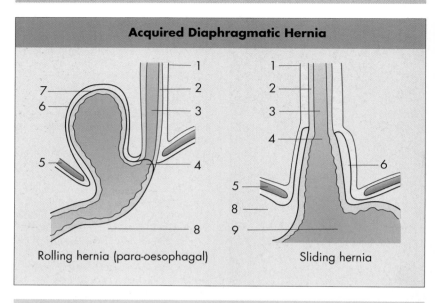

Acquired Diaphragmatic Hernia

Rolling hernia (para-oesophagal)

Sliding hernia

1	Pleura	6	Peritoneum
2	Oesophageal wall	7	Gastric wall
3	Oesophageal lumen	8	Peritoneal cavity
4	Oesophago-gastric junction	9	Gastric lumen
5	Diaphragm		

17.4 Acquired diaphragmatic hernia. Diagrammatic representation of the two principal types of hiatus hernia. A **sliding hiatus hernia** is common (95% of cases) whereas **para-oesophageal/rolling hiatus hernia** is rare. **Combined hiatus hernias**, in which there are both sliding and rolling components, are exceptional.

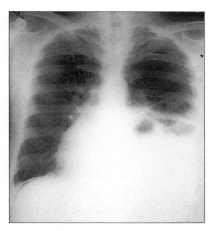

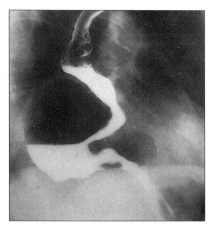

17.5 Rolling hiatus hernia. The chest radiograph shows a thoracic fluid level indicative of gastric contents within a herniated stomach. As intra-abdominal pressure normally exceeds intra-thoracic pressure, herniation of the stomach upwards is facilitated. Any additional increase in intra-abdominal pressure (straining, coughing and in pregnancy) favours herniation. Provided the lower oesophageal sphincter remains competent, there is no gastro–oesophageal reflux.

17.6 Sliding hiatus hernia. The barium swallow outlines the hernia, most of which is in the chest. The majority of patients are asymptomatic and the condition is frequently discovered coincidentally during upper gastro–intestinal radiology or endoscopy. Reflux oesophagitis produces the cardinal symptom of **heartburn**. This occurs soon after meals, is often promoted by stooping or recumbency, and is relieved by antacids. Water brash and reflux of fluid into the pharynx and mouth may also be present.

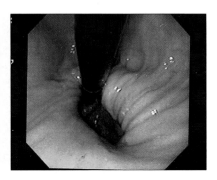

17.7 Sliding hiatus hernia: positive bell sign. The intra-thoracic cardia is viewed by the retroflexed endoscope giving the appearance of a church bell.

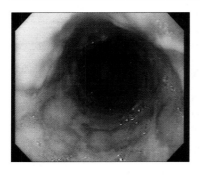

17.8 Grade IV oesophagitis.
Endoscopic features of oesophagitis with marked inflammation and ulceration of the mucosa in a symptomatic patient. The majority of patients can be managed medically with antacids, prokinetic agents, and H_2-antagonists or proton-pump blockers, depending on the degree of symptoms. Few patients require surgical intervention, the aim of which is to restore 'normal' anatomical relationships and to prevent gastro–oesophageal reflux.

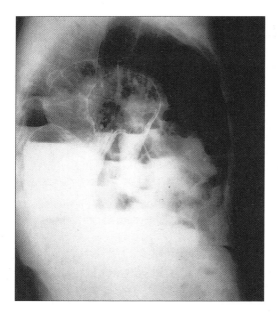

17.9 Traumatic diaphragmatic hernia. The lateral chest radiograph during a barium meal and follow-through shows bowel in the thoracic cavity following a missed diaphragmatic rupture. In 10% of patients with a fractured pelvis, traumatic rupture of the diaphragm may occur secondary to a sudden increase in intra-abdominal pressure following the crush injury to the pelvis. The diaphragmatic injury may go unrecognised initially until the patient presents with signs and symptoms related to the incarcerated/ strangulated organ or viscus (as shown). Penetrating chest or abdominal trauma can also breach the diaphragm.

Section 5

Abdomen

18.

THE ACUTE ABDOMEN

Abdominal pain is one of the most common symptoms to require investigation in the surgical patient. The onset, severity, localisation, radiation, precipitating and relieving factors, and any change in the character of pain, may aid diagnosis. Back pain caused by pathology involving retroperitoneal nerves may be the principal source of pain associated with diseases affecting the gallbladder, pancreas, duodenum or a ruptured aortic aneurysm. It is important to appreciate that perception of abdominal pain is relayed by the autonomic (visceral pain) and somatic (somatic pain) nervous systems.

VISCERAL PAIN

Visceral pain may be caused by excessive contraction or distension of a hollow viscus such as the intestine, ureter or gallbladder. It may also be evoked by localised ischaemia. Its nature is dull and deep-seated, and though it cannot be precisely localised it does bear relationship to the embryological origins of the primitive gut (**18.1**).

SOMATIC PAIN

The parietal peritoneum lining the abdominal wall is sensitive to tactile, thermal and chemical stimuli such as bile, intestinal content and blood. Stimulation results in sharp and highly localised somatic pain. There is associated overlying protective muscle guarding, rigidity and hyperaesthesia.

Associated Symptoms
Anorexia, **nausea** and **vomiting** are common symptoms in patients with acute abdominal pain. **Alteration in bowel habit**, particularly with the presence of **mucus, blood** or **melaena**, is usually indicative of serious pathology. In menarchal and pre-menopausal women it is important to ascertain the date of the **last menstrual period**, its normality, and the presence of other vaginal bleeding or discharge. Sexual history, oral contraceptive pill usage and the presence of dysmenorrhoeic symptoms may clarify a gynaecological aetiology. Mid-menstrual cycle pain, particularly in young girls (*Mittleschmerz*) is common, as the follicle

ruptures 14 days after the start of the last menstrual period and this may be complicated by bleeding causing lower abdominal pain.

Physical Signs

- **Inspection:** movement with respiration, abnormal pulsation or peristalsis, skin marking, and swellings in the flank or groin areas.
- **Palpation:** elicit site of pain and any associated guarding or tap tenderness, the presence of masses, or organomegaly (liver, spleen, kidneys and bladder).
- **Percussion:** for organomegaly and the presence of ascitic fluid.
- **Auscultation:** bowel sounds can be normal, increased, decreased or absent. Bruits are listened for over the abdominal aorta, and the renal, iliac and femoral vessels.
- **Rectal examination** is an integral part of the examination and a search is made for any obvious tenderness, masses or mucosal lesions.

Signs may be minimal in patients with dementia, in the elderly, patients on steroid therapy, the obese or the gravely ill. They may be masked in patients who have been sedated or given opiate analgesia.

Further Diagnostic Investigations

A full blood count, urea and electrolytes, liver function tests, amylase and glucose may be indicated. Prudent radiology including chest radiography and a plain supine abdominal radiograph may be helpful in determining the presence of supra-diaphragmatic pathology presenting as acute abdominal pain, pneumo-peritoneum, calculi and intestinal obstruction. The judicious use of intestinal contrast media, computer assisted tomography, ultrasonography, intravenous urography and angiography will be discussed in subsequent chapters.

Localisation of Visceral Pain

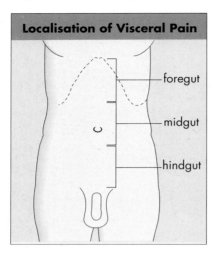

foregut

midgut

hindgut

18.1 Localisation of pain derived from the embryological gut. As the primitive gut was a midline structure, visceral pain is referred to the midline even though anatomical sites of organs are to the left or right. Organs with their embryological origin from the **foregut** (stomach, spleen, pancreas, liver, gallbladder) have visceral pain related to the epigastrium; from **midgut** structures (second part of the duodenum to the mid-transverse colon) to the peri-umbilical region; and from **hindgut** structures (distal transverse colon to the upper anal canal) to the suprapubic area.

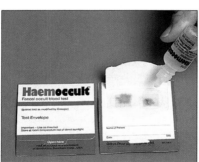

18.2 Faecal occult blood. The presence of faecal blood is indicated by the presence of a deep blue colour on the card of the haemoccult test.

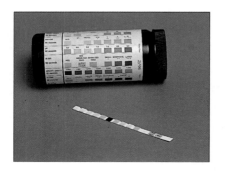

18.3 Urinalysis. The urinary dipstix may provide vital clues to the origin of abdominal pain or ongoing pathology. From left to right, each of the square patches tests for the presence of urobilinogen, protein, nitrite, pH, blood (highly positive in this patient), specific gravity, ketone, bilirubin and glucose. Microscopic examination of the urine may reveal pus cells and bacteria in urinary tract infections, and red blood cells in patients with renal colic.

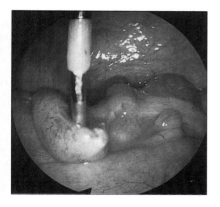

18.4 Diagnostic laparoscopy. This was carried out in a 16-year-old girl presenting with lower abdominal pain and an irregular menstrual cycle. Laparoscopy demonstrated acute appendicitis. There has been a rapid expansion in the use of both diagnostic and operative laparoscopy in recent years. Laparoscopy may afford accurate diagnosis and biopsy of tissue, and allow accurate intervention either as an open or laparoscopic procedure.

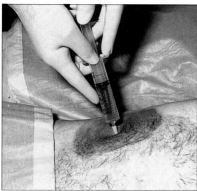

18.5 Fine-needle aspirate cytology. Elevation of white cell count, or the presence of bacteria on microscopy of peritoneal fluid obtained by lavage, may be indicative of abdominal pathology. Similarly, aspiration of ascitic fluid for bacteriological culture, biochemical analysis and microscopy for malignant cells is a useful adjunctive investigation.

ABDOMINAL ABSCESSES

Intra-abdominal abscesses are less frequent complications of surgery, due to antibiotic prophylaxis and improvements in surgical technique and instrumentation. Abscess development may follow elective surgery or result from inadequate lavage and cleansing of the peritoneal cavity where a viscus has perforated. The two common types of abscess formation are subphrenic and pelvic.

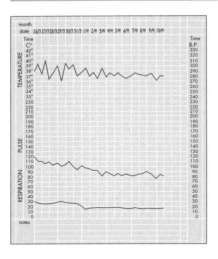

18.6 Pyrexia associated with intra-abdominal abscess formation.
This temperature chart shows a swinging pyrexia which began five days following a low anterior resection. The patient developed signs of systemic sepsis, heralded by tachycardia, pyrexia and an elevated white cell count. Anastomotic leakage was confirmed by gastrograffin enema and the presence of a pelvic abscess diagnosed by transabdominal ultrasonography.

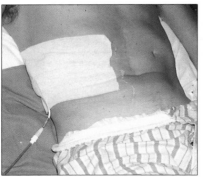

18.7 Percutaneous drainage of a subphrenic abscess.
This patient developed a subphrenic abscess following perforation of a peptic ulcer which had been managed conservatively. The subphrenic collection was drained percutaneously under ultrasound guidance. Chest radiography demonstrated a reactive right pleural effusion. Percutaneous drainage of intra-abdominal collections may be associated with damage to the bowel, bladder and major vessels.

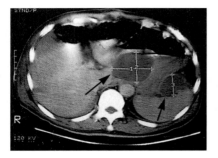

18.8 CT scan of intra-abdominal abscesses.
CT scanning is a useful adjunct to ultrasonography for delineating the size and site of intra-abdominal collections or for determining the presence of others not detected by ultrasound. This CT scan demonstrates two separate collections in the lesser sac and at the splenic hilus (arrows). Both abscesses were successfully drained by percutaneous means.

19.

STOMACH AND DUODENUM

Over the last decade, gastro–duodenal surgery has been undertaken less frequently, due to the falling incidence of gastric carcinoma and peptic ulceration coupled with improved medical therapy for the latter. It is therefore important to recognise the presence of gastro–duodenal pathology when it arises, and to investigate and treat the patient appropriately.

The **cardinal symptoms and signs** suggestive of gastro–duodenal disease include dyspepsia, nausea, vomiting, anorexia, weight loss or gain, regurgitation, haematemesis, melaena, localised abdominal tenderness, an epigastric mass, or systemic signs of malignancy such as cachexia, cutaneous manifestations or associated lymphadenopathy.

Diagnosis

- General examination and faecal occult blood.
- Full blood count, serum biochemistry and liver function tests.
- Upper gastrointestinal endoscopy with or without biopsy/brushings.*
- CLOtest for *Helicobacter pylori* (HP).
- C^{14} urea breath test for HP eradication.
- Chest radiograph.
- Barium meal.
- CT scanning.*
- Acid secretion studies.
- Gastro–intestinal hormone assays.
- Gastric emptying.
- Endoluminal ultrasonography.*
- Laparoscopy and laparoscopic ultrasonography.*

* *if tumour suspected*

The **mainstay of diagnosis** for most lesions of the upper GI tract is **endoscopic examination and biopsy** by an experienced endoscopist. Examination is not complete unless the second part of the duodenum is reached so that obvious duodenal pathology is not missed.

PYLORIC STENOSIS

Although **infantile hypertrophy** of the circular pyloric muscle causes **pyloric stenosis**, the underlying pathogenesis of this condition is poorly understood. Eighty per cent of instances occur in male infants, 50 per cent of cases are first-born infants, and the condition occurs more frequently in siblings. The infant usually presents 4–6 weeks after birth and rarely after 12 weeks of age. The presenting symptom is projectile vomiting which does not contain any bile. The infant takes food avidly immediately after vomiting but there is failure to thrive, dehydration and constipation. **Ramstedt's pyloromyotomy** is the standard surgical treatment, splitting the circular muscle to allow the mucosa to bulge through the defect. The infant returns to normal feeding a few hours after surgery.

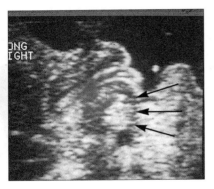

19.1 Congenital hypertrophic pyloric stenosis. 75% of cases have a palpable pyloric 'tumour' which is felt as a firm, peanut-sized swelling in the epigastrium or right upper quadrant, during a test feed when the child is relaxed. Where there is doubt regarding the diagnosis, contrast study or trans-cutaneous ultrasonography (as shown) usually demonstrates the pyloric 'tumour' (arrows). Consider in the **differential diagnosis** enteritis, neonatal intestinal obstruction, cranial birth injury and over-feeding.

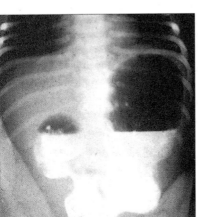

19.2 Duodenal atresia. This contrast study is diagnostic as it shows distension of the stomach and the proximal duodenum with absence of gas throughout the rest of the bowel. Vomiting in this condition occurs from birth and the stomach is visibly distended. Duodenal atresia may be caused by a complete absence of the duodenum, a fibrous band, a diaphragm or stenosis. There is a high incidence of trisomy 13.

PEPTIC ULCERATION

Peptic ulceration results from an imbalance between gastric secretion and the ability of the mucosa of the upper GI tract to withstand peptic digestion. Excessive or inappropriate acid and pepsin secretion is implicated in duodenal ulceration, whereas hypersecretion is not of primary importance for the development of gastric ulceration. Defective mucosal defences are thought to be the principal factor leading to ulceration in patients with normal or reduced secretion capacity. However, ulceration does not occur in the absence of acid and pepsin secretion.

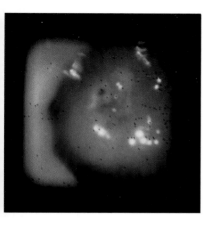

19.3 Chronic duodenal ulcer. Endoscopic examination demonstrated a posterior ulcer in the first part of the duodenum of a 28-year-old male who presented with a 12-month history of intermittent epigastric pain. His symptoms were episodic, occurring every 3–6 months and lasting 7–10 days. His dyspepsia was relieved within minutes of taking food and wakened him during the night between 2 and 3 o'clock in the morning. Prepyloric ulcers behave like their duodenal counterparts but biopsy is mandatory as a small percentage may be early gastric cancers.

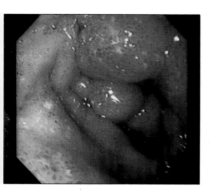

19.4 Duodenitis. This 50-year-old male, who smoked 20 cigarettes a day and consumed in excess of 30 units of alcohol a week, complained for many years of intermittent dyspepsia relieved by antacids. Biopsy of the antral mucosa demonstrated antral gastritis and *H. pylori* organisms. He responded to eradication therapy, omeprazole and a change in his lifestyle.

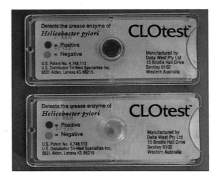

19.5 CLOtest for *H. pylori*. A positive test is indicated by the presence of a pink colour change. Various regimens exist for eradication therapy (e.g., triple therapy consisting of amoxycillin 500 mg 8-hourly. and metronidazole 400 mg 8-hourly. for 2 weeks; and omeprazole 20 mg once a day for 4 weeks). Eradication of the organism is checked by C^{14} breath test.

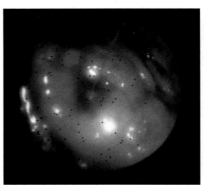
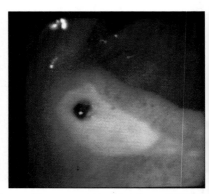

19.6 Bleeding duodenal ulcer. This 65-year-old woman, taking diclofenac (NSAID) for osteoarthritis of the hip, presented with a large haematemesis and hypovolaemic shock. Emergency endoscopy demonstrated an actively bleeding posterior ulcer in the first part of the duodenum (*left*). Bleeding from duodenal ulcers will cease in 90% following injection of 1 in 100,000 adrenaline. Rebleeding is more likely to occur in larger ulcers (greater than 1 cm in diameter) and where there is a visible vessel present (*right*).

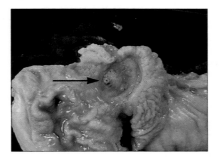

19.7 Bleeding duodenal ulcer – postmortem specimen. Despite advances in both the endoscopic and surgical treatment of bleeding peptic ulcer, the overall mortality has changed little in recent years. This postmortem specimen is of a patient who was not successfully resuscitated following a massive haematemesis. A large duodenal ulcer has eroded through the gastroduodenal artery (arrow).

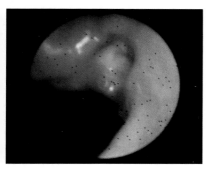

19.8 Chronic gastric ulcer.

Endoscopy shows a chronic gastric ulcer with evidence of recent haemorrhage on the lesser curvature at the incisura. This is usually associated with gastritis and develops at the junction between the acid secreting and non-acid secreting mucosa. Endoscopic biopsy is mandatory, with repeat endoscopy to ensure treatment response. Non-healing of any ulcer demands repeat biopsy and mucosal brushings.

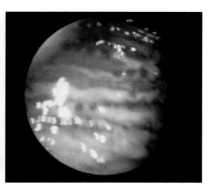

19.9 Acute gastric erosions. This

68-year-old woman with peripheral vascular disease and carotid bruits had been commenced on enteric-coated aspirin 300 mg per day. A small haematemesis precipitated admission and endoscopy demonstrated acute gastric erosions caused by the aspirin. She reponded to cessation of aspirin and simple antacid therapy. **Other causes of gastric erosions** include: NSAIDs, stress (following surgery, trauma, burns) and excessive biliary reflux.

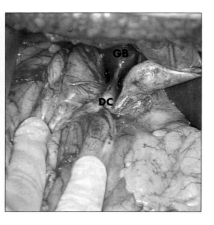

19.10 Chronic duodenal

ulceration. At operation a grossly scarred duodenal cap (DC) is seen, to which the gallbladder (GB) and liver were densely adherent. During the polya gastrectomy the ulcer base posteriorly was left on the pancreatic parenchyma. All peptic ulcers resistant to treatment (including eradication therapy) should be investigated for a hormonal source such as gastrinoma and Zollinger–Ellison syndrome.

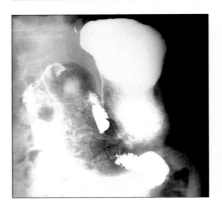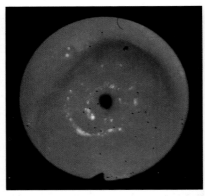

19.11 Acquired pyloric stenosis. The barium meal (*left*) shows a massively dilated stomach due to a severely scarred pylorus. Note the metal clips at the oesophageal hiatus from a previous vagotomy. Endoscopy confirms a pinhole pylorus (*right*). Her presentation was of weight loss, heartburn and recurrent vomiting of foodstuffs 2–3 days-old. There were signs of dehydration, cachexia and a marked **succussion splash** indicative of fluid retention within the stomach.

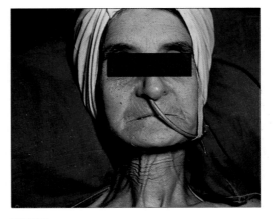

19.12 Acquired pyloric stenosis. This patient presented with pyloric stenosis and nutritional depletion with a serum albumin of 21 g/l. She was sustained on total parenteral nutrition for three weeks with her albumin rising to 32 g/l prior to surgery (vagotomy and gastro-enterostomy) and 37 g/l prior to discharge.

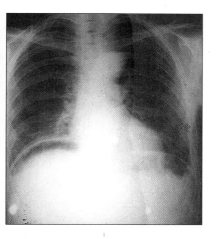

19.13 Pneumoperitoneum. Chest radiograph of a young man with a known peptic ulcer who presented with sudden onset of severe epigastric pain. Only 70% of perforated duodenal ulcers will give rise to a pneumoperitoneum and, if the diagnosis is suspected and no free air seen, a gastrograffin swallow may demonstrate a leak. **Differential diagnosis** includes: other perforated viscera, laparotomy, laparoscopy, penetrating trauma, peritonitis due to gas-forming organisms, and gynaecological investigations. The patient underwent suturing of an omental patch and oversew of the perforation.

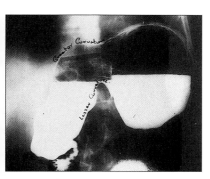

19.14 Gastric Volvulus. The barium meal shows organo-axial volvulus of the stomach. The presentation may be acute, causing gastric strangulation and infarction or, as in this patient, symptoms may be intermittent, requiring elective investigation.

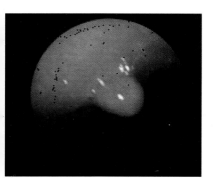

19.15 Gastric polyposis. Adenomatous polyps are the most common benign neoplasms to arise from the epithelium and may be single or multiple. The risk of malignant transformation increases with polyp size and with multiplicity. These lesions are often found incidentally on barium meal examination or endoscopy (as shown), but can give rise to bleeding or intermittent pyloric obstruction with vomiting.

CARCINOMA OF THE STOMACH

Classification of Gastric Neoplasms

Benign

- Adenomatous polyp.
- Leiomyoma.
- Neurogenic tumour.
- Fibroma.
- Lipoma.

Malignant

- Adenocarcinoma.
- Lymphoma.
- Leiomyosarcoma.

The stomach is the second most common site for cancer of the gastro–intestinal tract. In the UK each year, 50–60 people per 100,000 population are affected by the disease which accounts for 10 per cent of cancer deaths. The five-year survival rate is still less than 10 per cent.

Risk Factors

Males; increasing age (1 in 15 cases occur in patients under 40 years of age); genetic (first-degree relatives with the disease); blood group A; geographic (higher incidence in Japan, South America and Eastern Europe than in the UK or North America); atrophic gastritis; pernicious anaemia; adenomatous polyps; previous gastrectomy; chronic gastric ulceration; unskilled social group; occupation (miners, rubber and asbestos workers); and diet (nitrate salts).

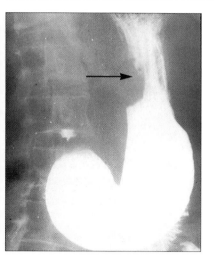

19.16 Leiomyoma. The most common mode of presentation is haematemesis. Leiomyomas account for approximately 2% of all upper GI bleeds due to ulceration. The submucosal location of the lesion makes it difficult to obtain a representative endoscopic biopsy. The contrast examination shows the typical appearances of a 4 cm lesion situated on the lesser curve of the stomach (arrow). Although some would suggest local resection of such lesions, it is difficult to establish their malignant potential and a more radical approach may be justified.

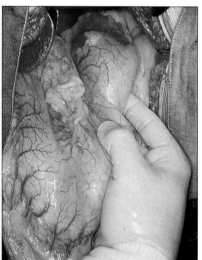

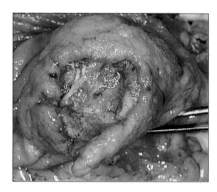

19.17 Leiomyosarcoma of the fundus. This patient presented with weight loss and anaemia. Endoscopy found an ulcerated mucosal lesion which was malignant on biopsy. At operation the 6 cm lesion was easily palpable at the fundus and upper lesser curve (**left**). A total gastrectomy was performed for the ulcerated lesion which is seen on the opened specimen (**right**).

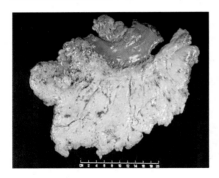 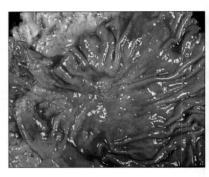

19.18 Antral carcinoma. Distal radical gastrectomy for cancer (*left*). Endoscopic biopsy of a chronic gastric ulcer, which had not healed on medical treatment, had shown dysplastic change. Subsequent histological examination confirmed malignancy of the raised ulcer (*right*).

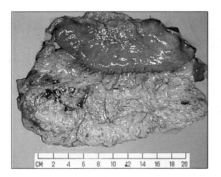 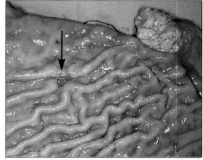

19.19 Early gastric cancer (EGC). Distal radical gastrectomy for EGC (*left*). The opened specimen shows a small ulcer (*right*) which had been shown by endoscopic biopsy to be malignant and by endoluminal ultrasound to be confined to the submucosa. In the UK, less than 5% of all gastric neoplasms present in this manner, although if selected populations are targeted for screening, the detection rate for EGC increases to 25%.

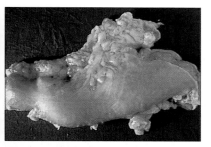

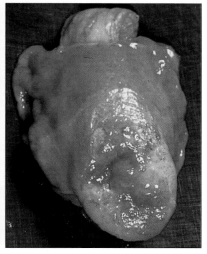

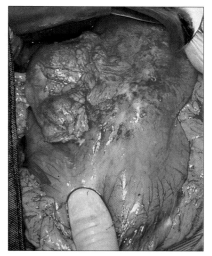

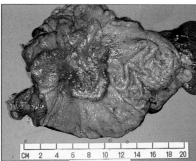

19.20   Linitus plastica. This pathological specimen (***top***) demonstrates the infiltrative nature of the gastric cancer in a 66-year-old male who presented with anorexia, 22 kg weight loss and anaemia. His stomach was rigid at endoscopy. The gastric cross-section shows a grossly thickened 'leather bottle' wall (***bottom***). Four months later he developed enlargement of the left supraclavicular nodes due to spread along the thoracic duct (**Troisier's sign**).

19.21   R2 gastric resection. This operative photograph shows an infiltrative carcinoma of the mid-stomach with extensive lesser curve nodal involvement (***top***). An R2 gastric resection (total gastrectomy and splenectomy with coeliac lymphatic clearance) was performed. A large ulcerating lesion is seen in the opened specimen (***bottom***).

20.

LIVER

The **signs and symptoms** that become evident with the presence of liver disease are due to **disturbance** of **normal anatomy** or **physiology**. The liver is comprised of hepatic lobules formed by sheets of hepatocytes which are separated by venous sinusoids. These drain blood from the portal venous system to the central branches of the hepatic venous system. Bile is secreted by the hepatocytes and small canaliculi which pass through the lobules into bile ductules leading to the principal left and right hepatic ducts.

Diagnosis
- General examination.
- Full blood count and coagulation screen.
- Serum biochemistry, total protein, albumin.
- Liver function tests: alkaline phosphatase, gamma GT, AST, ALT, bilirubin.
- Serology: autoantibodies, hepatitis and other viral infections, amoebic and hydatid.
- Liver biopsy.
- Chest radiograph.
- Ultrasonography: transcutaneous, laparoscopic, intra-operative.
- CT scanning: enhanced, iodised oil emulsion, portography.
- Sulphur–colloid scanning.
- Magnetic resonance imaging.
- Angiography: coeliac, mesenteric, trans-splenoportography.
- Laparoscopy.

HEPATOMEGALY

Principal Differential Diagnosis of Hepatomegaly
- Infection: viral hepatitis, liver abscess, protozoal infestation.
- Primary and secondary neoplasia.
- Cystic disease: single/multiple.
- Disorders in metabolism.
- Autoimmune.
- Normal: diaphragmatic depression from emphysematous lungs, Reidle's lobe.

Segmental Liver Anatomy

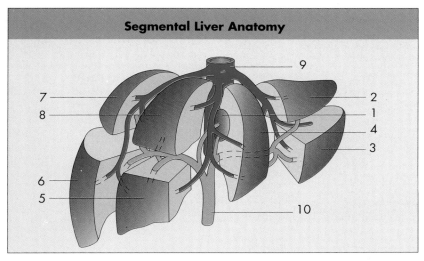

20.1   Liver anatomy. Anatomically, the left and right hemi-livers are marked by an imaginary line drawn from the gallbladder fossa to the inferior vena cava, although, for descriptive purposes, the right and left lobes lie to either side of the falciform ligament. The liver normally receives 1500 ml of blood per minute and has a dual supply: 65% comes from the portal vein and 35% from the hepatic artery. The left, middle and right hepatic veins drain posteriorly into the inferior vena cava.

1–8	Liver segments
9	Inferior vena cava
10	Portal vein

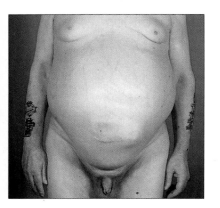

20.2   Systemic signs of liver disease. This 55-year-old patient had a long history of chronic alcohol abuse and developed cirrhosis of the liver. Jaundice, gynaecomastia, testicular atrophy, loss of pubic hair, gross ascites and hepatomegaly are present.

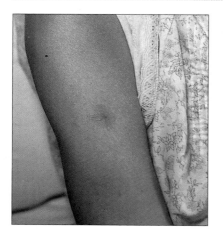

20.3   Systemic signs of liver disease. In this 32-year-old female, the signs of liver disease are much more subtle: mild clinical jaundice and spider naevi as shown on the upper half of her body. Isolated spider naevi are not pathological in themselves and do not require any specific treatment.

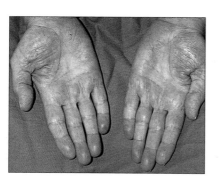

20.4   Hand signs of chronic liver disease. This patient with end-stage liver disease exhibits palmar erythema, early Dupuytren's contracture and clubbing. Leuconychia (white nails) and a flapping tremor were also present.

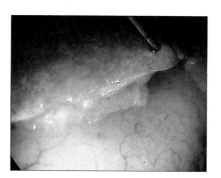

20.5   Laparoscopic liver biopsy. Liver biopsy using a trucut needle is carried out under direct vision by laparoscopy, using local anaesthesia and low pressure insufflation of the abdominal cavity (8 mmHg) with nitrous oxide. Prior to carrying out liver biopsy, it is important that a platelet count and coagulation screen have been carried out.

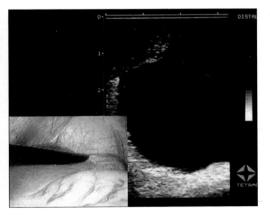

20.6 Simple hepatic cyst. This laparoscopic hepatic ultrasonograph confirms the characteristic anechoic features of a 5 cm simple cyst in segment 2. Simple liver cysts are present in 40% of the population, rarely give rise to symptoms, and should be differentiated from polycystic and hydatid disease of the liver. In this patient the roof of the symptomatic cyst was excised by laparoscopic means.

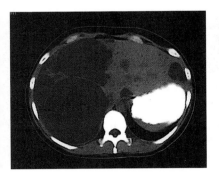
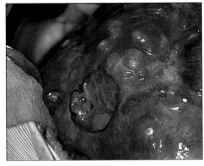

20.7 Polycystic liver disease. This CT scan shows multiple bilobar cysts replacing much of the parenchyma (**left**). This patient's liver function was normal. The principle symptom was that of abdominal distension and dragging discomfort. In this patient open surgery was undertaken to deal adequately with the posteriorly situated cysts (**right**). There is a high recurrence rate if cysts are decompressed by percutaneous means or if multiple small cysts are present.

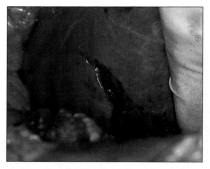

20.8 Penetrating hepatic trauma.
This 18-year-old male was a victim of a stabbing assault, in which he sustained a number of penetrating wounds to the abdomen and back resulting in profound hypovolaemic shock. At emergency laparotomy, there was a deep laceration of the right lobe of the liver. Even if the entry wound is remote from an abdominal organ, a major intra-abdominal injury should be suspected in a patient presenting with hypovolaemia.

20.9 Blunt hepatic trauma: angiography.
This angiogram shows an arterio–portal venous fistula (arrowed) and an extensive contusion in the right lobe of the liver following blunt abdominal trauma. This patient did not require surgery and settled on conservative measures.

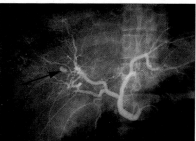

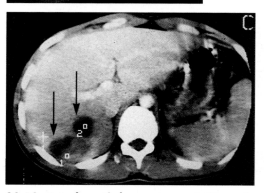

20.10 Intrahepatic haematoma. A CT scan in a 40-year-old pedestrian knocked down by a bus, sustaining a right-sided blunt abdominal trauma, shows an extensive intrahepatic haematoma. The principle risks are of continued expansion and sudden disruption of the liver parenchyma with resultant catastrophic and fatal haemorrhage. This type of blunt injury differs from a deceleration injury, in which the right lateral sector (segments 6 and 7) is disrupted by the shearing force exerted along the liver's attachment to the diaphragm by the right triangular ligament.

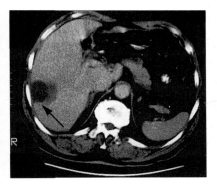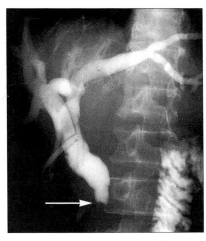

20.11 Hepatic abscess. Hepatic abscesses may be bacterial, parasitic or fungal.
The bacterial abscess is more common in the Western world, but parasitic infestation is
an important cause worldwide. In this patient's CT scan, a solitary right lobe abscess
(*left*) is caused by recurrent cholangitis due to impaired drainage of the bile duct and
retained stones (*right*). Treatment was by by percutaneous drainage of the abscess,
antibiotic therapy and endoscopic removal of the calculi.

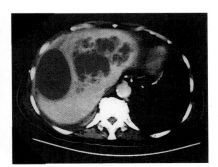

20.12 Multiple pyogenic abscesses. This liver CT scan shows multiple abscesses
caused by diverticulitis. Bacterial infection has arisen in this instance via the **portal**
system but can also gain access from the **biliary** system, by the **hepatic artery** from a
septic focus at a distant site and by **direct spread** such as empyema of the gallbadder.
In approximately half the cases, the abscess is **cryptogenic** and no cause can be
found. The most common infecting organisms are Gram negative bacteria, notably
Streptococcus milleri and *Escherichia coli*.

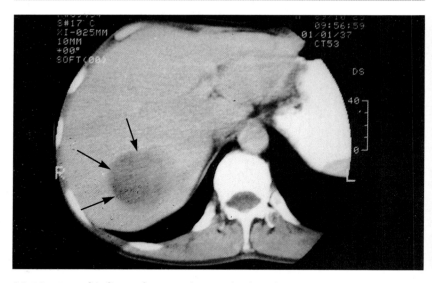

20.13 Amoebic liver abscess. These tend to be solitary and situated in the right lobe, and may reach sizeable proportions. The abscess contains brownish pus resembling anchovy sauce. A CT scan was performed in a patient complaining of right upper quadrant (RUQ) pain, anorexia, weight loss and nocturnal sweats, with tender liver enlargement (present in over 90% of patients with this condition). The scan shows a typically poorly delineated collection. The abscess is caused by a protozoal parasite, *Entamoeba histolytica*, which infests the large intestine and is endemic in many tropical regions. This patient had recently returned from South-East Asia, where he had been working for several years. Amoebic cysts were found in stool samples by microscopy. Serology also detects amoebic protein antigens. This patient was treated with metronidazole resulting in rapid resolution.

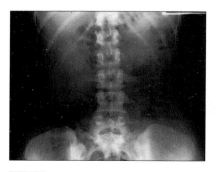

20.14 Hydatid cyst. This calcified lesion seen in the RUQ of a Shetland farmer on plain abdominal radiography is due to a hydatid cyst. These cysts are caused by *Echinococcus granulosus/multilocularis*, an adult tape worm living in the dog intestine whose intermediate hosts are sheep and man. The condition is common in sheep rearing areas such as Australia, Greece and the Western Isles of Scotland.

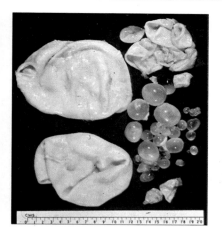

20.15 Hydatid cysts. These pathological specimens are the main cysts and their daughter cysts following surgical excision from the liver. Spillage of contents at surgery can lead to anaphylactic reactions and the dissemination of viable scolices. At operation, contamination is avoided by isolation of the operating field with packs, aspiration of the cyst contents and application of a scolicidal agent such as hypertonic saline or 0.5% silver nitrate. Mebendazole is an alternative to surgical treatment but its value remains uncertain.

PORTAL HYPERTENSION

Normal portal pressure is 4–8 mmHg. When there is **increased resistance to flow** through the portal venous circulation, portal pressure rises and portal hypertension ensues, despite the development of portocollateral circulation. Alternatively, increased portal pressure may result from **increased blood flow** through the portal circulation, but this is rare.

Principal Causes of Portal Hypertension

Pre-hepatic
- Congenital portal vein atresia.
- Portal vein thrombosis: umbilical sepsis in neonates, appendicitis/diverticulitis in adults and older children.
- Extrinsic portal vein compression.

Intrahepatic
- Cirrhosis: alcoholic, viral, primary biliary, cryptogenic.
- Schistosomiasis (*Bilharzia Mansonii*).

Post-hepatic
- Budd–Chiari syndrome.
- Constrictive pericarditis.

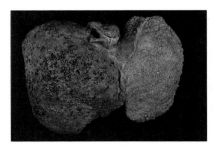 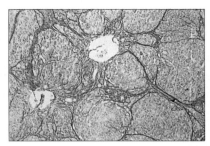

20.16 Micronodular cirrhosis. Cirrhosis is the most common cause of portal hypertension (*left*), the aetiology of which is predominantly alcohol in the Western world, schistosomiasis in North Africa and the Middle East, and chronic active hepatitis secondary to hepatitis B in South-East Asia, Central and Southern Africa. Progressive hepatocyte damage, fibrosis and nodular regeneration reduce the space of Disse, resulting in elevated resistance to flow and increased portal pressure (*right*).

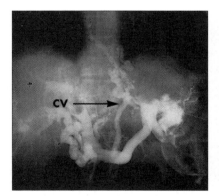 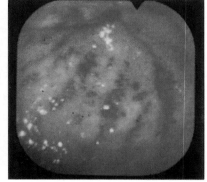

20.17 Porto–systemic collateral circulation. Raised portal pressure is the driving force leading to the development of porto-collateral shunts. This is clinically important at the oesophago–gastric junction, in the retroperitoneal and peri-umbilical areas and in the anorectal venous plexus. The trans-splenic portal venogram shows an extensive porto-systemic collateral circulation in the venous phase of the examination (*left*). Note the prominent oesophago–gastric varices filling from the coronary vein (CV). Increased blood flow through the gastric submucosal plexus may cause marked telangiectasia (portal hypertensive gastropathy, *right*).

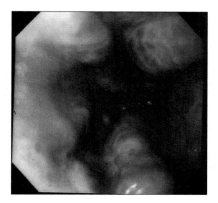 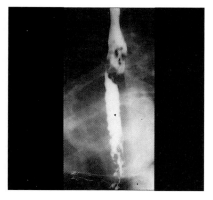

20.18 Oesophageal varices. Large varices with red spots (wale markings) are at high risk of rupture and catastrophic variceal haemorrhage (**left**). Prophylactic intervention is tempting when varices are detected incidentally, as in this barium swallow (**right**). Currently, there is no evidence that prophylactic injection sclerotherapy, variceal banding or porto-systemic shunt surgery have any beneficial effect on mortality before the index bleed, although propranolol or nadolol reduce or delay the onset of the initial variceal bleed.

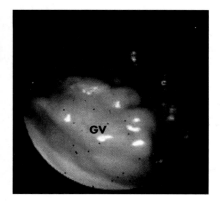 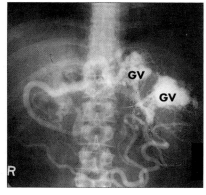

20.19 Gastric varices. They should be suspected in patients with known portal hypertension presenting with upper GI bleeding in whom an obvious cause (oesophageal varices or peptic ulceration) is not readily evident. Isolated gastric varices (GV) are found high on the posterior fundic wall (**left**). They are associated with substantial gastro–renal shunts and located in the fundus (**right**).

NEOPLASMS OF THE LIVER

Classification of Liver Neoplasms

Benign
- Cavernous haemangioma.
- Adenoma.
- Focal nodular hyperplasia.

Malignant
- Hepatocellular carcinoma.
- Cholangiocarcinoma.
- Hepatoblastoma.
- Angiosarcoma.
- Metastases.

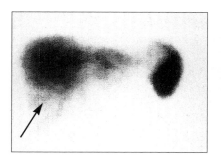 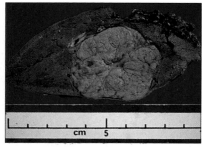

20.20 Fibronodular hyperplasia. This 24-year-old female patient presented with vague dyspeptic symptoms and was shown to have a lesion in the right hemi-liver and had normal liver function tests. The isotope scan has unusually demonstrated a filling defect in the tip of the right lobe of the liver (***left***). The lesion was resected because of the uncertainty of the underlying pathology but the transected specimen shows the typical central scar and lobulated appearance of fibronodular hyperplasia (***right***).

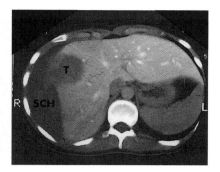 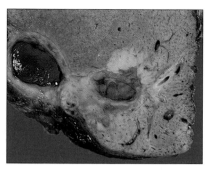

20.21 Hepatic adenoma. Adenomas are commonly asymptomatic but this patient presented with acute abdominal pain and collapse from a spontaneous bleed from this vascular lesion. The CT scan shows subcapsular haematoma (SCH) but the tumour (T) is not easily seen (**left**). The haemorrhage settled spontaneously and resection was undertaken three months later (**right**). Adenomas are resected because they are often symptomatic, may bleed and may undergo malignant change. The role of the oral contraceptive pill in their development is not well understood.

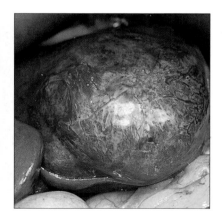 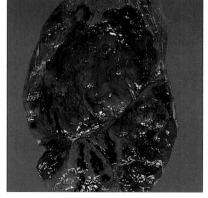

20.22 Hepatocellular carcinoma. This operative picture shows a vascular hepatoma occupying the left lobe of the liver in a 26-year-old man (**left**). The diagnosis was confirmed by a markedly raised alphafetoprotein. If hepatoma is suspected and surgical resection is under consideration, trucut biopsy or fine-needle aspiration should not be performed, in order to avoid the risk of bleeding and the dissemination of tumour. The cut specimen shows a well-differentiated hepatoma in a non-cirrhotic patient (**right**).

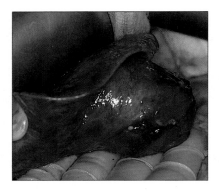

20.23 Hepatoma. One of the characteristics of hepatoma is their vascular nature. Approximately 10% of patients with hepatoma present with a rupture of the lesion and catastrophic peritoneal haemorrhage. This patient had a small hepatoma on the undersurface of the left lobe which had presented in this way. Dissemination of tumour cells into the peritoneal cavity is inevitable. Tumours can spread via the portal vein branches, to regional lymph nodes and to lung and bone.

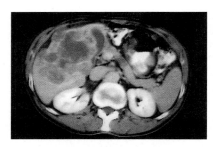

20.24 Hepatoma. This patient presented with right upper quadrant pain and an abdominal mass which, on CT scan, is seen to occupy almost all the entire right lobe of the liver (**top**). The alphafetoprotein levels were normal and there were no obvious aetiological factors evident. Because there was no underlying cirrhosis an extended right hepatic resection was undertaken (**middle**) and the postoperative scan on the seventh postoperative day shows massive hypertrophy of the residual left lobe (**bottom**).

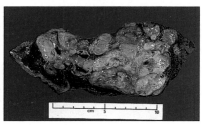

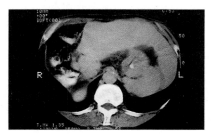

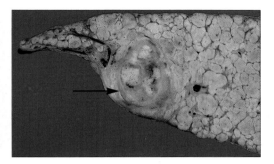

20.25 Hepatoma. This pathological specimen shows a small hepatoma removed by means of a segmental resection to avoid liver failure in this cirrhotic patient. In patients with non-resectable disease, alternative treatments include direct injection with absolute alcohol, chemo-embolisation, cryotherapy or laser ablation. Hepatoma is the most common male cancer worldwide. It is uncommon in the Western world but is predominant in Africa and the Far East. The principal aetiology is Hepatitis B surface antigen carriage, although in Africa, aflatoxin derived from the fungus *Aspergillus flavus* and contaminating maize and nuts is an important hepatocarcinogen. Viral hepatitis is a preventable disease by Hepatitis B vaccination.

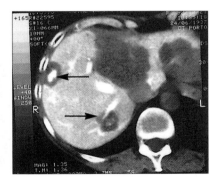

20.26 Colorectal hepatic metastases. CT arterial portography is widely regarded as the best means of delineating metastatic disease within the liver. The diagnosis can be confirmed by elevation of the carcinoembryonic antigen and, if necessary, fine-needle aspiration or trucut biopsy where surgery is not being contemplated. This patient had previously been treated by embolisation of the tumour and the lipiodol can be seen to have been retained by the two metastases in the right lobe. Two further rapidly expanding lesions are evident on the left side. Alternative treatments of colorectal metastases include systemic chemotherapy, intermittent hepatic artery ischaemia, regional chemotherapy by means of an indwelling hepatic artery catheter, laser ablation and cryotherapy. Selected patients may be suitable for resection.

21.

GALLBLADDER AND BILE DUCTS

The **cardinal symptoms and signs** of gallbladder disease are: right upper quadrant (RUQ) pain, fatty food intolerance, nausea, vomiting and, occasionally, jaundice, associated with RUQ tenderness, muscle guarding and a mass. Biliary colic is a pain present in the epigastrium and across the upper abdomen as the gallbladder contracts against stones in Hartmann's pouch. RUQ pain may radiate through to the back between the scapulae and to the right shoulder.

Diagnosis

- General examination.
- Urinalysis.
- Full blood count and prothrombin time.
- Liver function tests.
- Ultrasonography.
- Oral cholecystography.
- Intravenous cholangiography.
- Technetium[99] HIDA scanning.

If jaundice present:

- Endoscopic retrograde cholangiopancreatography (ERCP).

- Percutaneous trans-hepatic cholangiography (PTC).

If malignancy suspected:

- Biliary cytology.
- CT scanning.
- Laparoscopy.

Anatomy of the biliary system

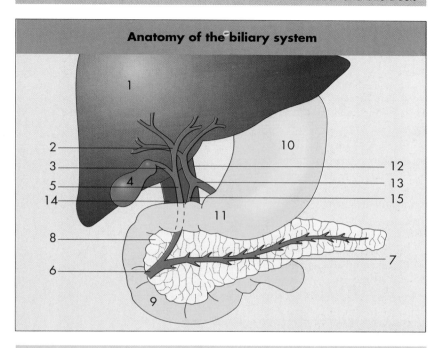

1	Liver	9	Duodenum
2	Common hepatic duct	10	Body of stomach
3	Cystic duct	11	Antrum
4	Gallbladder	12	Portal vein
5	Common bile duct	13	Hepatic artery
6	Ampulla of Vater	14	Inferior vena cava
7	Pancreatic duct	15	Gastroduodenal artery
8	Head of pancreas		

21.1   Anatomy of the biliary system. Intrahepatic biliary radicals form the left and right hepatic ducts which converge in the porta hepatis to form the common hepatic duct. This duct joins the cystic duct to form the common bile duct, which terminates at the ampulla of Vater where it is joined by the main pancreatic duct. The gallbladder lies in a fossa on the undersurface of the liver between the anatomical right and left lobes. It consists of a fundus, a body and a neck which is usually supplied by the right hepatic artery via the cystic artery, which passes posterior to the cystic duct. Hartmann's pouch is a dilatation of the gallbladder outlet adjacent to the origin of the cystic duct and in which gallstones frequently become impacted. Considerable variation in biliary anatomy exists.

JAUNDICE

Principal Differential Diagnosis of Obstructive Jaundice

Lumen
- Choledocholithiasis.
- Stent blockage.
- Parasitic infection, e.g. ascariasis.

Wall
- Benign tumours of the biliary tree.
- Peri-ampullary carcinoma.
- Cholangiocarcinoma.
- Post-traumatic or infective cholangitis stricture.
- Sclerosing cholangitis.

Extrinsic
- Carcinoma of the pancreas.
- Mirizzi's syndrome.
- Portal lymphadenopathy.
- Locally invasive cancers.

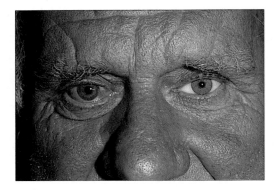

21.2 Jaundice. This patient with obstructive jaundice has clear evidence of hyperbilirubinaemia. He has an artificial left eye, which aids in the detection of discoloration of the sclera, an early sign of jaundice. Clinically apparent jaundice should be evident at 50 μmol/l (normal range 15–22 μmol/l). **Obstructive jaundice** causes pale stools and dark urine (urinary dipstix will indicate large amounts of conjugated bilirubin and no urobilinogen). The bilirubin will be elevated, together with the alkaline phosphatase and gamma GT.

CONGENITAL ABNORMALITIES

The gallbladder is derived from a diverticulum which grows out from the ventral wall of the foregut. It differentiates into the hepatic duct and the liver. The lateral bud from this diverticulum becomes the gallbladder and the cystic duct. Congenital abnormalities of the gallbladder and bile ducts are common.

DEVELOPMENTAL ABNORMALITIES

- Congential absence of the gallbladder or cystic duct.
- Duplication.
- Intrahepatic partition with a fold in the fundus.
- Multiple septate gallbladder.
- Long mesentery to the gallbladder.
- Biliary atresia.
- Choledochal cysts.

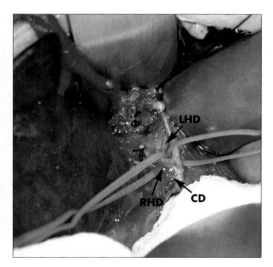

21.3 Biliary atresia. This operative slide shows the atretic left (LHD) and right hepatic ducts (RHD) forming the common duct (CD), after cholecystectomy in a neonate presenting with obstructive jaundice and hepato-splenomegaly three weeks postnatally. Atresia occurs in 1 in 20,000–30,000 births. The principal **differential diagnosis** is neonatal hepatitis. Surgical treatment is by means of a Roux-en-Y anastomosis to the biliary remnants at the porta hepatis (**Kasai operation**). The failure to recognise this condition leads to progressive cirrhosis, hepatic failure and death. Liver transplantation may offer the only hope of survival.

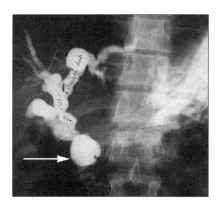

21.4 Choledochal cyst. This very thin patient presented with intermittent pain, jaundice and attacks of pancreatitis. A mass was palpable in the right hypochondrium. ERCP demonstrated marked dilatation of the extrahepatic bile ducts. The cyst was resected because of the significant risk of malignant transformation. The biliary tree was reconstructed by hepatico– jejunostomy Roux-en-Y.

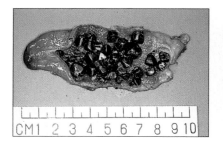 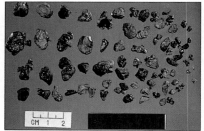

21.5 Cholelithiasis. Cholecystectomy for gallbladder stones is the most common major surgical procedure carried out throughout the world, and is now performed by laparoscopic means (**left**). The incidence of gallstone disease increases with age and can occur in at least 20% of women over the age of 40. The incidence in males is about one-third of that in females. The three principal types of stone are mixed, pure cholesterol and bile pigment stones (**right**).

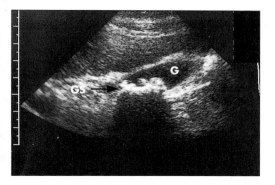

21.6 Gallbladder ultrasonography.

Ultrasonography has replaced oral cholecystography as the principal means of diagnosing the presence of stones. The ultrasonogram shows multiple stones in the gallbladder (G) with characteristic acoustic shadows behind the stones (GS).

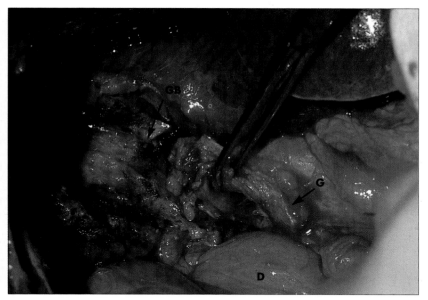

21.7 Acute cholecystitis. This patient presented with acute epigastric and RUQ pain, tenderness in the subcostal margin at the tip of the 9th rib (Murphy's sign), and pyrexia. Surgery is best undertaken during the same admission but, in this patient, laparoscopic cholecystectomy was abandoned because of the dense inflammatory reaction around the gallbladder (G) and surrounding liver. Acute cholecystitis is usually caused by obstruction of the neck of the gallbladder or cystic duct by a stone. Complications of acute cholecystitis include empyema and gangrene of the gallbladder, and perforation. GB = gallbladder bed; D = duodenum.

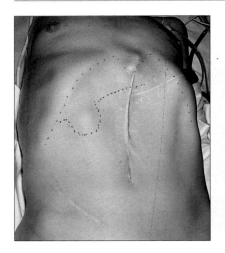

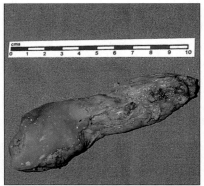

21.8 Mucocele of the gallblader. This patient presented with intermittent RUQ pain which became worse after meals. The gallbladder is visible in the RUQ and was readily palpable (***left***). The patient has had a number of operations for complications of peptic ulcer disease and this previous history has probably contributed to the development of his gallstones. The opened specimen contained small calculi and pale mucus (***right***).

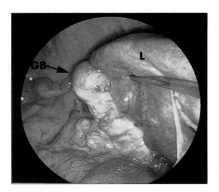

21.9 Chronic cholecystitis. This laparoscopic view shows the most common form of symptomatic gallbladder (GB) disease. It is almost invariably associated with gallstones and characterised by RUQ pain and fatty food intolerance. The gallbladder is small, fibrotic and contracted. L = liver.

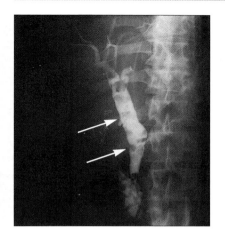

21.10   Operative cholangiography.
This cholangiogram shows marked dilation
(13 mm) of the common bile duct, within
which are numerous calculi. 10% of
patients undergoing cholecystectomy have
choledocholithiasis, although the
cholangiogram is useful in defining the
anatomy during a difficult cholecystectomy.

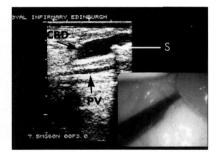

**21.11   Laparoscopic
ultrasonography of biliary tree.**
Laparoscopic ultrasonography allows
visualisation of both the intra-hepatic and
extra-hepatic biliary tree and is a possible
alternative to cholangiography. Using the
linear array probe, the common duct is
followed caudally to demonstrate acoustic
shadowing within the dilated common bile
duct (CBD) due to calculi.
S = stone; PV = portal vein.

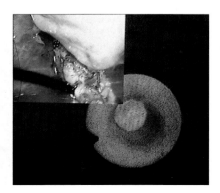

**21.12   Laparoscopic trans-cystic
duct exploration.** In this patient, stones
were seen on both laparoscopic ultrasound and operative cholangiography.
The common bile duct has been explored
with a 5 mm choledochoscope via the
cystic duct. The stones were successfully
extracted and clearance of the duct was
achieved. A tube can be left in the cystic
duct to allow postoperative cholangiography so as to confirm the clearance of
the common bile duct.

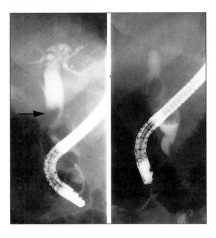

21.13 ERCP. The cholangiogram in this patient confirms the presence of stones which were missed at laparoscopic cholecystectomy because a cholangiogram was not undertaken (**far left**). Following sphincterotomy and Dormier basket extraction the stones appear through the papillotomy (**near left**).

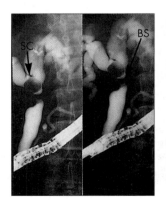

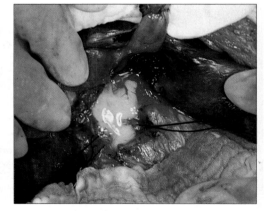

21.14 Choledocholithiasis and cholangitis. This patient presented with fever, rigors, jaundice and RUQ pain (Charcot's triad). This episode of cholangitis necessitated emergency ERCP which shows a solitary calculus (SC) proximal to a benign stricture (BS) (**left**). Opening the common hepatic duct, there was instant release of pus (**right**). Intrahepatic choledocholithiasis is a common problem in South-East Asia.

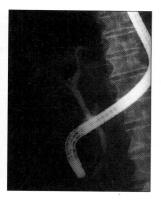
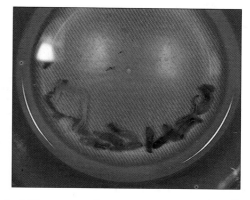

21.15 Parasitic infestation of the biliary tree. The ERCP (***left***) shows filling defects in the lower CBD which could not be cleared. Exploration of the common duct was performed and multiple *Clonorchis senensis* organisms were extracted (***right***). Multiple irrigations post-operatively via T-tube drainage remove most parasites. Systemic therapy using praziquantel eradicate the rest.

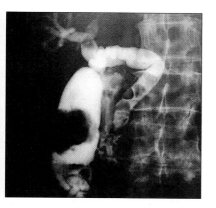
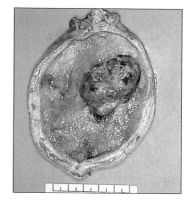

21.16 Carcinoma of the gallbladder. This is rare and almost invariably related to the presence of gallstones (***left***). It is four times as common in females as in males. 90% of the lesions are adenocarcinomas, the remainder are squamous cell carcinomas. 'Cure' may only be possible if a small tumour has been found incidentally on the non-gallbladder fossa side during the removal of a gallbladder for stone disease (***right***). Trisigmentectomy and regional lymph node dissection may improve prognosis. The five-year survival rate in Western countries is 5%. In Japan, five-year survival rates of up to 30% have been reported.

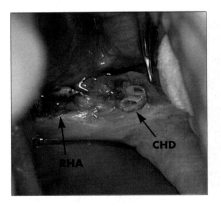

21.17 Common bile duct injury.
This patient presented with severe abdominal pain and signs of generalised peritonitis 48 hours after her cholecystectomy. The injury was unrecognised at the time of laparoscopic cholecystectomy. The common bile duct had been resected and the right hepatic artery (RHA) was divided and ligated. On the right of the picture, the divided cystic and common hepatic ducts (CHD) are clearly seen. Repair was instituted using hepatico–jejunostomy Roux-en-Y.

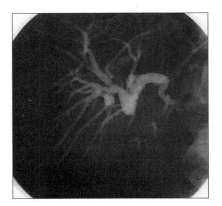

21.18 Benign biliary stricture.
Cholangiography demonstrates a stricture of the common hepatic duct two years after a difficult open cholecystectomy had been carried out. The patient had presented with recurrent attacks of acute cholangitis and was at risk of developing secondary biliary cirrhosis. This type of injury is ischaemic in nature and secondary to excessive use of diathermy or extensive clearing of the common duct. Repair was instituted using hepatico–jejunostomy Roux-en-Y.

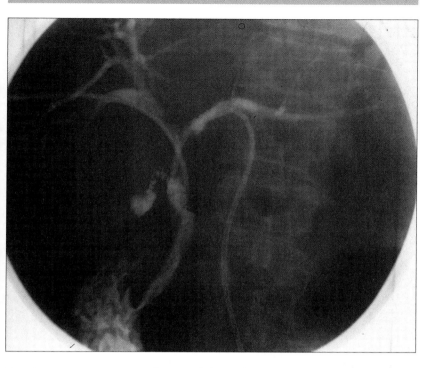

21.19 Percutaneous transhepatic biliary drainage of a
cholangiocarcinoma. Cholangiocarcinoma is a relatively uncommon lesion which affects the elderly, but it may be increasing in frequency. It may arise from the extrahepatic or intrahepatic bile ducts, or their confluence (**Klatskin tumour**) as shown here. It may be difficult to differentiate from sclerosing cholangitis. Percutaneous transhepatic cholangiography and biliary drainage allow diagnosis of the obstructing lesion. The procedure is therapeutic by stenting the obstructing lesion in the patient not considered for resection. Percutaneous cytological brushings following transhepatic biliary drainage may confirm the presence of a cholangiocarcinoma. Alternatively, these brushings may be obtained by endoscopic retrograde cholangiography and brush biopsy, although this has a variable success rate.

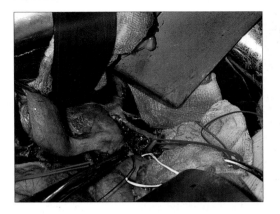

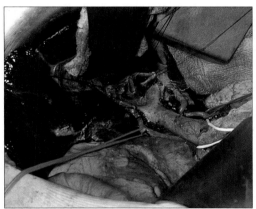

21.20 Cholangio-carcinoma. The common bile duct will be dissected along with the lymphatic tissues and the gallbladder from the portal vein (white sling) and the left and right hepatic arteries (red and blue slings) (**top**). The right hepatic artery has an aberrant origin from the superior mesenteric artery, an abnormality which occurs in 20% of individuals. Once the extrahepatic biliary tree has been resected the portal vein and its branches can be seen (**bottom**). The hepatic ducts are anastomosed to a Roux-en-Y limb of jejunum. Resection, possible in less than 20% of patients, offers the only prospect of survival.

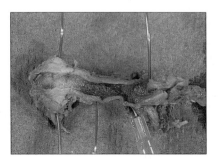

21.21 Pathological specimen of a Klatskin tumour. This shows the diffuse infiltrative nature of the lesion which requires that frozen section of the left and right hepatic ducts is performed to ensure that clearance of the tumour has been obtained. Cholangiocarcinomas may be diagnosed incidentally in recipients' livers which are removed in preparation for transplantation for primary sclerosing cholangitis.

22.

PANCREAS

The pancreas develops as a dorsal and ventral bud from the duodenum. The ventral bud rotates posteriorly, enclosing the superior mesenteric vessels, and forms the major part of the head of the pancreas drained by the main duct of Wirsung. In most patients the duct of Wirsung has a common opening with the common bile duct (CBD) in the ampulla of Vater. The dorsal bud becomes the body and tail of the pancreas and its duct becomes the accessory duct of Santorini. The CBD passes through the head of the pancreas, and obstructive jaundice is frequently due to neoplasia or inflammation involving this part of the gland.

The development of **symptoms and signs** depends on whether the pathophysiological process affects the function of the exocrine or endocrine pancreas, or both. Upper abdominal pain arising from the pancreas is invariably poorly localised to the epigastrium and radiates through to the back. It may be severe in acute pancreatitis, and is of a gnawing nature in pancreatic cancer. Vomiting, steatorrhoea, weight loss, jaundice and an epigastric mass may be presenting features of pancreatic disease. Late-onset diabetes may be an early sign of pancreatic disease but pancreatic endocrine hyperfunction may present with such bizarre symptoms as hypoglycaemia, personality disorder or skin rash.

Diagnosis

- General examination.
- Full blood count and prothrombin time.
- Liver function tests, amylase, glucose, total protein, albumin.
- Chest radiograph.
- Ultrasonography: transcutaneous, laparoscopic, intra-operative.
- Endoscopic retrograde cholangiopancreatography (ERCP).
- Percutaneous transhepatic cholangiography (PTC).

If neoplasia suspected:
- Biliary cytology.
- Hormonal assays.
- CT scanning.
- CT-guided fine-needle aspiration.
- Angiography.
- Laparoscopy.

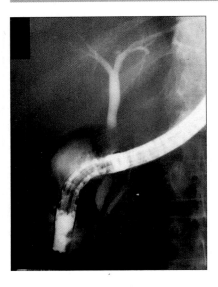

22.1 Pancreas divisum. The pancreatogram shows failure of fusion of the ducts draining both components of the pancreas. This anatomical variation occurs in approximately 5% of individuals. The physiological significance is that most of the pancreatic secretions ascend into the duodenum through the small accessory duct. Its pathological significance is not certain, but it has been a suggested cause of both acute and chronic pancreatitis.

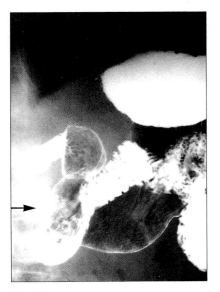

22.2 Annular pancreas. This barium meal intake and follow through shows a collar of pancreatic tissue surrounding the second part of the duodenum producing an obstruction. It is caused when the two developmental buds envelop the second part of the duodenum in conjunction with failure of the ventral bud rotation posteriorly. Accessory budding from the primitive foregut occurs in 20% of individuals with heterotropic pancreatic tissue which may be found in the stomach, duodenum or jejunum.

ACUTE PANCREATITIS

Aetiology

In the UK, there are between 50 and 100 new cases of acute pancreatitis per million population each year. All adult age groups may be affected. Acute pancreatitis carries a risk of morbidity and mortality of approximately 10 per cent.

Principal causes
- Gallstones (40%).
- Alcohol (40%).
- Idiopathic (15%).

Other causes
- Pancreatic cancer (4%).
- Drugs (steroids, diuretics).
- Renal transplantation.
- Hyperlipidaemia.
- Hyperparathyroidism.
- Viral infection (mumps, Coxsackie B, cytomegalovirus, Epstein–Barr).
- Hypothermia.
- Polyarteritis nodosa.
- Scorpion bites.
- Pregnancy.
- Previous polya gastrectomy.
- Trauma (operative, blunt, penetrating).
- Investigation (ERCP or arteriography).

Differential Diagnosis
- Perforated peptic ulcer.
- Acute cholecystitis.
- Ruptured aortic aneurysm.
- Myocardial infarction.
- Spontaneous rupture of the oesophagus.
- Pericarditis.

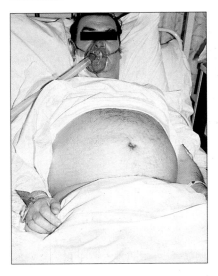

22.3   Acute pancreatitis. This patient, suffering from a severe attack of acute pancreatitis, presented with a recent history of excess alcohol intake, severe epigastric pain radiating through to his back, repeated vomiting and retching. Clinical examination demonstrated hypotension with tachycardia, a left pleural effusion, abdomen distension with tenderness, guarding and rigidity in the epigastrium. Haematological and biochemical predictors of severity of disease were: elevated white blood cell count 17,000, glucose 13.6 mmol/l, corrected calcium 2.01 mmol/l, albumin 28 g/l, and pO_2 7.2 kPa. His amylase was elevated to 3000 IU/L but this in itself is not a predictor of severity of disease.

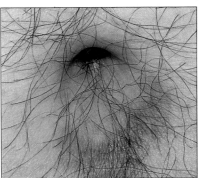

22.4   Cullen's sign. The haemorrhagic discoloration around the umbilicus is usually indicative of haemorrhagic pancreatitis, although in itself it is rare. It is usually due to the products of pancreatic necrosis tracking along the falciform and umbilical ligaments.

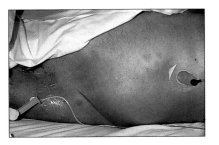

22.5   Grey Turner's sign. This is not dissimilar to Cullen's sign but the discoloration is present in the loins due to tracking of pancreatic necrotic material along the retroperitoneal planes. Both these signs are markers of a severe insult to the pancreas.

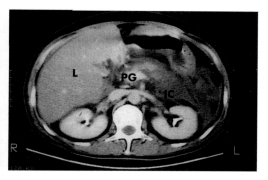

22.6 Contrast-enhanced CT scan of acute pancreatitis. This scan in a 40-year-old woman with gallstone-related pancreatitis shows marked oedema of the whole of the pancreas gland (PG) with the typical 'smoke and fire' appearance of inflammatory changes (IC) in the surrounding tissues, in particular the mesentery extending to the left para-colic gutter. Intravenous contrast enhancement shows necrotic areas within the pancreas. Ultrasound scanning early in the presentation of acute pancreatitis is useful in delineating the presence of gallstones, bile duct dilatation, pancreatic oedema, fluid collections and even the presence of pleural effusions. L = liver.

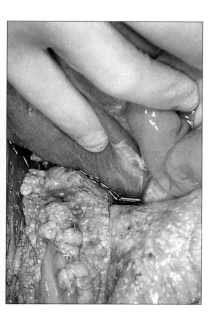

22.7 Acute pancreatitis with fat necrosis. Surgery was undertaken in this patient who continued to deteriorate clinically and had a rising C-reactive protein (30.3 mg/l), which is usually indicative of pancreatic necrosis. The CRP is one of the best markers of the progress of the disease. The operative view shows widespread fat necrosis present within the mesentery and omentum causing the speckling appearance of fat and contributing to the hypocalcaemia associated with this condition.

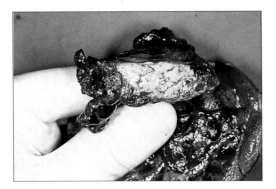

22.8 Peri-pancreatic necrosis. Pancreatic necrosectomy was carried out together with debridement of necrotic retroperitoneal tissue which necessitated distal pancreatectomy and splenectomy. The cut section margin of the pancreas shows relatively normal internal pancreatic tissue and evidence of the characteristic peri-pancreatic necrosis.

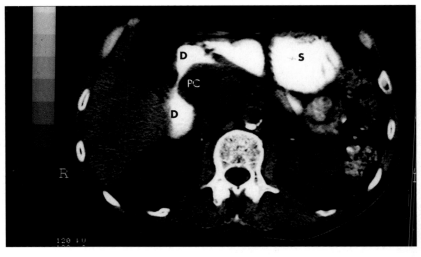

22.9 Pseudocyst of the pancreatic head. This CT scan shows a mature pseudocyst (PC) indenting the duodenum (D) some 8 weeks after the initial episode of acute pancreatitis. A pseudocyst is a collection of pancreatic secretions and inflammatory exudate within the lining of inflammatory tissue and is located in the lesser sac or retroperitoneal tissue around the pancreas. Pseudocysts usually occur in 10% of patients following alcohol or traumatic pancreatitis. Small cysts are often asymptomatic and resolve spontaneously. If the cysts have failed to resolve on follow-up ultrasonography by 6 weeks, they are unlikely to do so without intervention. Larger collections, such as the one shown, displace and compress the stomach or duodenum causing considerable discomfort. Persistent elevation of the serum amylase may also be indicative of the presence of a pseudocyst. S = stomach; L = liver.

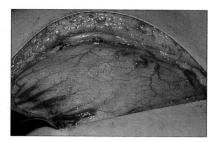

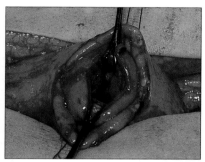

22.10 Pseudocyst in the lesser sac. This large pseudocyst is seen to be pushing the stomach forwards at operation (**top**). Although double pigtail catheters can be inserted between stomach and cyst cavity, the most effective means of cyst drainage is surgical, usually by a pseudocyst gastrostomy (**bottom**) or jejunostomy Roux-en-Y. Untreated, pseudocysts are at risk of abscess formation, obstructive jaundice, persistent duodenal ileus and severe haemorrhage.

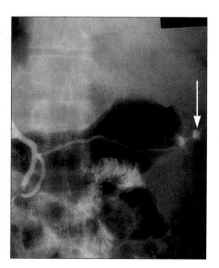

22.11 Pancreatic fistula. This endoscopic retrograde pancreatogram demonstrates leakage of contrast into the left upper quadrant (LUQ) from a distal pancreatic duct following a splenectomy for trauma. Persistent clear fluid drainage from an LUQ tube drain had an amylase content of 235,000 IU/l indicative of the presence of pancreatic fistula. This patient was managed by intravenous nutritional support for 4 weeks and administration of subcutaneous octreotide.

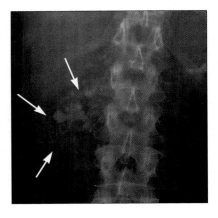

22.12 Chronic pancreatitis. This abdominal radiograph demonstrates marked LUQ calcification. This 35-year-old patient with a long-standing history of alcoholism presented with an 8 kg weight loss, steatorrhoea and marked pain precipitated by eating, spreading through to his back and eased by bending forwards. Although alcoholism is the most common aetiological factor, cholelithiasis may be present in 25% of patients. Malnutrition, mucoviscidosis, hyperparathyroidism, haemochromatosis and familial pancreatitis are more rare causes of this condition.

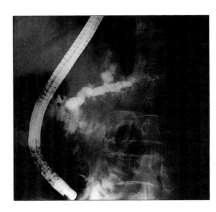
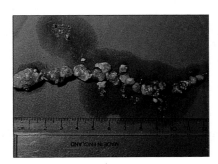

22.13 Chronic pancreatitis. The pancreatogram shows the disrupted architecture of the pancreatic duct at ERCP (**top**). The chronic inflammation leads to progressive replacement of the gland by fibrous tissue, destroying ductal and islet tissue. Multiple strictures form in the pancreatic duct, further impairing drainage. Protein plugs form in the ducts and later calcify. **Principles of management**: remove the aetiological agent (alcohol or gallstones), replace functional deficiencies of both exocrine and endocrine function, and alleviate pain. Surgery may be indicated to manage intractable pain and includes pancreatico–jejunostomy, Whipple's procedure, distal pancreatectomy and total pancreatectomy. In this patient a pancreatico–jejunostomy has been performed after removal of the pancreatic duct calculi (**bottom**).

PANCREATIC NEOPLASMS

Pancreatic carcinoma is increasing in frequency, and is now the fourth most common cause of cancer death in males and the sixth most common in females in many Western countries. Men are more frequently affected than women and the peak incidence is between 55 and 70 years of age. Risk factors include tobacco smoking and a diet high in both fat and protein.

Classification of Pancreatic Neoplasms

Benign exocrine
- Peri-ampullary villous adenoma.
- Pseudo-cystadenoma.
- Mucinous cystadenoma.

Malignant exocrine
- Adenocarcinoma.
- Cystadenocarcinoma.
- Invasion from carcinoma of the stomach or cholangiocarcinoma.

Endocrine
- Insulinoma.
- Glucagonoma.
- Vipoma.
- Somatostatinoma.

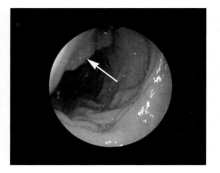 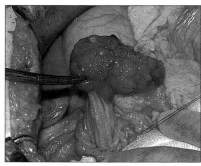

22.14 Peri-ampullary cancer. This demonstrates the importance of reaching the second part of the duodenum where a peri-ampullary lesion (11 o'clock) was detected incidentally during investigation for gastro–oesophageal reflux in a 72-year-old woman (**left**). Endoscopic sphincterotomy or stent insertion may be considered in the unfit patient. A transduodenal approach was used to excise the ampullary lesion locally (**right**) in this patient, rather than a Whipple's resection.

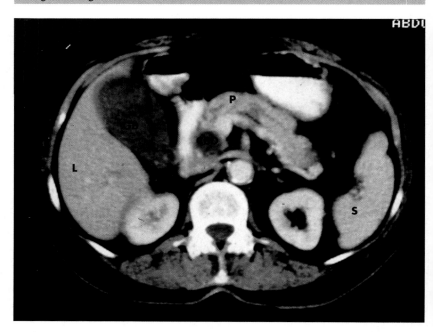

22.15 Pancreatic cancer – Couvoisier's law. This 55-year-old patient presented with a 3-month history of weight loss, anorexia, malaise, vomiting, deepening jaundice and gnawing epigastric pain. The CT scan revealed a distended gallbladder (GB) and a dilated common bile duct (CBD). Couvoisier's law states that, in the presence of jaundice, a palpable gallbladder is more likely to be due to an obstructing pancreatic neoplasm than to gallstones. A chronically inflamed gallbladder will probably be small and shrunken in the patient, with jaundice due to gallstones unless a mucocele is present. L= liver; P = pancreas; S = spleen.

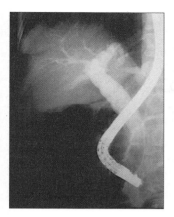

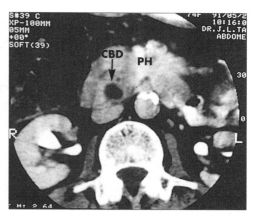

22.16 Pancreatic carcinoma. In a patient with obstructive jaundice ERCP demonstrated a stricture of the lower CBD (*left*). On CT scanning the pancreatic head (PH) was diffusely enlarged, CBD dilatation was marked and there was no overt evidence of metastatic disease (*right*). Although angiography determines the route map for variable arterial and portal venous anatomy, it provides little predictability of resection.

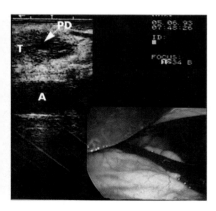

22.17 Laparoscopic ultrasonography of pancreatic carcinoma. This 56-year-old woman presenting with obstructive jaundice was judged to have irresectable carcinoma by conventional imaging methods. Laparoscopy was undertaken and did not demonstrate any evidence of peritoneal or hepatic dissemination. Laparoscopic ultrasonographic examination showed a tumour (T) measuring 3 cm in diameter, clear of the underlying portal vein. This patient underwent a pancreatico–duodenectomy. All lymph nodes examined were negative for nodal metastases. A = aorta; PD = pancreatic duct.

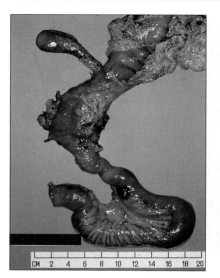
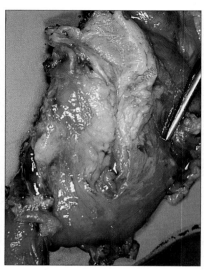

22.18 Carcinoma of the pancreas – Whipple's resection. By the time of presentation, few patients have tumours small enough to be considered both resectable and curative. Surgery involves resection of the stomach, pancreatic head and bile duct, gallbladder and duodenum (**left**). The common duct has been opened demonstrating the extrinsic compression by the pancreatic tumour (**right**).

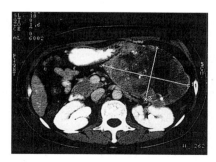
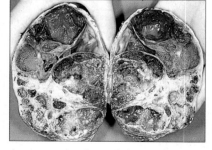

22.19 Cystadenoma. This 37-year-old male presented with weight loss, vomiting and epigastric fullness. Clinical examination confirmed the presence of a mass in the epigastrium in the left upper quadrant. CT scanning revealed a large cystic mass in the body and tail of the pancreas (**left**). The resected specimen (distal pancreatectomy and splenectomy) shows a large, multi-septate cystic mass (**right**). Histology confirmed its benign nature. These tumours are rare and smaller ones can be enucleated.

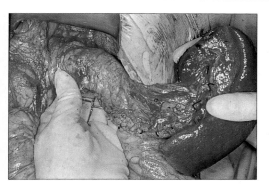

22.20 Insulinoma. The diagnosis of these lesions can be difficult as the presentation is very variable. Hyperinsulinaemia causes hypoglycaemic symptoms; if mild, these include intellectual and motor impairment with insidious personality changes; if severe, bizarre behaviour, sweating, palpitations and tremor may be found. Confirmation of the diagnosis of insulinoma depends on demonstrating hypoglycaemia (fasting blood glucose of <2.2 mmol/l) and excess insulin secretion. Multiple insulinomas occur usually as part of the multiple endocrine neoplasia syndrome. Therefore the whole gland must be examined by palpation and intra-operative ultrasound since pre-operative localisation can be difficult.

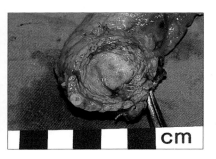

22.21 Insulinoma. Surgical removal of the tumour is the treatment of choice, although enucleation may be possible. Insulinomas arise from the beta cells of the islets of Langerhans and tend to be small and single. Most insulinomas (more than 90%) are benign.

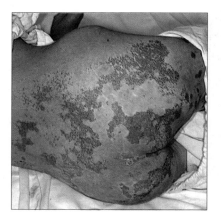

22.22 Glucagonoma: necrolytic migratory erythema. This characteristic rash presents over the buttocks, legs and arms. It had been treated by dermatologists for several months with a variety of topical applications without improvement. There was also painful angular stomatitis, diarrhoea, weight loss, diabetes mellitus and anaemia. The finding of an elevated glucagon in association with this rash is pathognomonic of a glucagonoma. The diagnosis was subsequently confirmed by elevated serum glucagon levels and a CT scan of the pancreas.

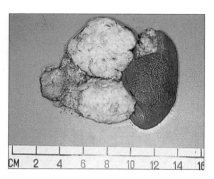

22.23 Glucagonoma. The resected specimen of the tail of the pancreas and spleen confirms the presence of a small glucagonoma.

23.

SPLEEN

Symptoms of splenomegaly relate to the underlying cause of the condition, originate from local compression of the adjacent structures or are due to splenic infarction with pleuritic left upper quadrant (LUQ) pain radiating to the left shoulder. The two principal **differential diagnosis** of a left upper quadrant mass are a renal mass and gastric neoplasia.

SPLENOMEGALY

Classification of Splenomegaly

Infections
- Viral: glandular fever.
- Bacterial: typhus, typhoid, septicaemia.
- Protozoal: malaria, kala-azar, schistosomiasis.
- Parasitic: hydatid.

Haemopoietic disease
- Leukaemia, Hodgkin's disease, non-Hodgkin's lymphoma.
- Pernicious anaemia, polycythaemia, myelofibrosis.

Portal hypertension
Metabolic and collagen diseases
- Amyloidosis, Gaucher's disease.
- Still's disease.

Miscellaneous
- Cysts, abscesses and splenic tumours (very uncommon).

Indications for Splenectomy
- Trauma (blunt or iatrogenic).
- Combined, as part of another operative procedure such as gastrectomy or pancreatectomy.
- Blood disorders: haemolytic anaemia, idiopathic/acquired thrombocytopenia.
- Tumours and cysts.

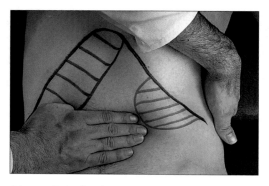

23.1 Clinical splenomegaly. The spleen is a friable, blood-filled organ lying in the left upper quadrant of the abdomen, protected by the 9th–11th ribs. It weighs about 150 g and lies with its long axis along the length of the tenth rib. The spleen must be enlarged two to three-fold before it becomes clinically palpable. It descends below the left costal margin towards the right iliac fossa, moves on respiration and has a firm lower margin which may or may not be notched. The mass is dull to percussion and the dullness extends above the costal margin.

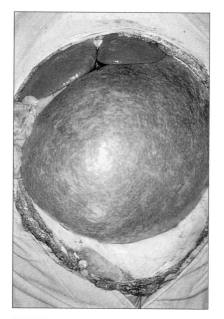

23.2 Myelofibrosis. This giant spleen, weighing 5.5 kg and occupying approximately 25% of the peritoneal cavity, was approached through an extended subcostal incision, and was removed for symptomatic reasons. Massive splenomegaly in Western countries is likely to be due to chronic leukaemia, lymphoma, polycythaemia or portal hypertension. If splenomegaly is found, a careful examination must be undertaken to detect associated hepatomegaly and lymphadenopathy.

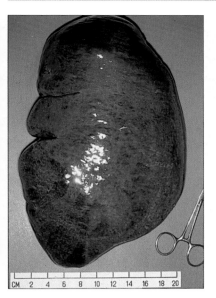

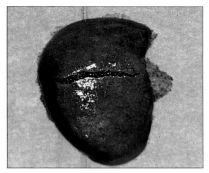

23.4 Splenic laceration. The specimen shows a major parenchymal laceration of the spleen due to a fractured left 10th rib, causing uncontrollable bleeding. Although a variety of spleen-conserving operations have been advocated, few are practical in the haemodynamically unstable patient; the development of fibrin tissue glues may offer more promise. The diagnosis of splenic injuries requires a higher degree of suspicion, as both ultrasound and peritoneal lavage can be misleading. Because of the susceptibility following removal to infections such as *pneumococcus, influenza* and *meningococcus*, there is a growing tendency to attempt conservative management of splenic injuries, particularly in children.

23.3 Hairy cell leukaemia.
Recurrent LUQ pleuritic pain due to multiple splenic infarctions precipitated splenectomy. Although the weight of the specimen was 4.8 kg, removal of the organ was aided by initial ligation of the splenic vessels which reduced its size (unlike in myelofibrotic spleens) by about 25%. Patchy discoloration is indicative of splenic infarct sites.

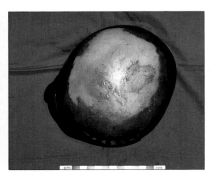

23.5 Splenic cyst. Cysts of the spleen are rare and usually single (multiple in polycystic disease). Single cysts may be **degenerative, parasitic** or, as in this particular patient, **congenital** which is secondary to an embryonic defect and results in a dermoid-like lesion. They are lined by flattened epithelium and contain thin blood-stained fluid or, in this case, thick creamy material. Usually these cysts are asymptomatic and are often discovered incidentally.

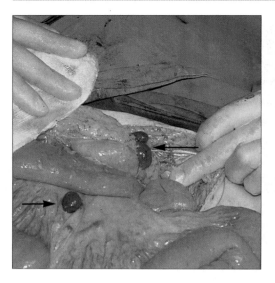

23.6 Idiothrombo-cytopenic purpura and splenunculi.

One of the most common indications for splenectomy is failure of steroid therapy to control idiopathic thrombocytopenia, a disease which is characterised by a low platelet count and a short platelet lifespan. Splenomegaly is unusual. However, it is vital to identify and remove splenunculi which may occur in the splenic hilum, the greater omentum – where three were found in this patient – and, rarely, in the small bowel mesentery as shown.

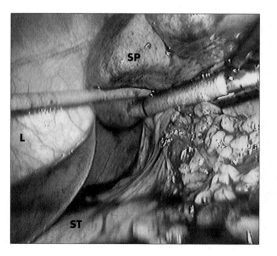

23.7 Acquired thrombocytopenia.

Patients with human immunodeficiency virus infection may develop marked thrombocytopenia. The spleen (SP) is usually of normal size but, to minimise the risk to theatre and ancillary staff, laparoscopic splenectomy in these individuals is now possible. The laparoscopic view shows an endoGIA vascular stapler across the splenic hilum. ST = stomach; L = liver.

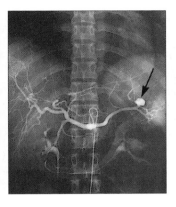
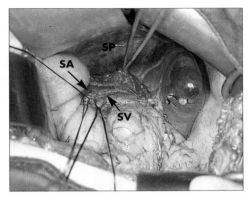

23.8   Splenic artery mycotic aneurysm. A patient with infective endocarditis developed intermittent LUQ pain. Coeliac axis arteriography demonstrated a splenic artery aneurysm (***left***) which was at risk of rupture. Control of the splenic artery (SA) and vein (SV) were essential prior to splenic pulp mobilisation (***right***). SP = spleen.

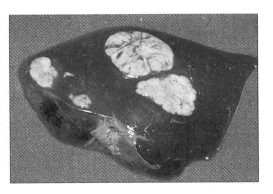

23.9   Metastatic melanoma. Secondary tumours in the spleen are rare but melanoma has a propensity to metastasise to unusual sites, often many years after the initial presentation.

24.

SPECIFIC AND SPECIAL FORMS OF OBSTRUCTION

Classification of Intestinal Obstruction

Level
- High or low small bowel.
- Colonic.

Onset
- Acute.
- Subacute.
- Chronic.
- Acute-on-chronic.

Pathological process
- Intra-luminal.
- Mural.
- Extra-mural.

The **cardinal symptoms and signs** of intestinal obstruction are: abdominal colic; vomiting which occurs early in high intestinal obstruction and late in low small bowel or colonic obstruction; relative (passage of flatus only) or absolute constipation (failing to pass either flatus or faeces); abdominal distension (although this may be absent in a high obstruction); visible peristalsis; and auscultation revealing obstructive, high-pitched and tinkling bowel sounds. **Localised pain, tenderness and guarding implies strangulation and demands urgent surgery.**

Volvulus is the rotation of a bowel loop around its mesenteric axis, which results in obstruction and occlusion of the main vessels at the base of the involved mesentery. It most commonly affects the sigmoid, caecum and small intestine, but volvulus of the gallbladder and stomach may also occur. The **precipitating factors** include abnormalities of intestinal loop mobility and length, the presence of adhesions to the loop apex and loops with a narrow pedicle.

Differential Diagnosis of Congenital Intestinal Obstruction

- Intestinal atresia or stenosis.
- Malrotation of the gut.
- Hirschsprung's disease.
- Meconium ileus.
- Imperforate anus.
- Acquired obstruction due to milk curds.

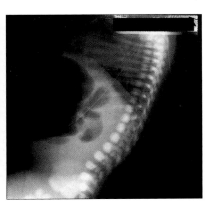

24.1   Ileal atresia. A supine abdominal radiograph is the most valuable investigation to diagnose the aetiology of intestinal obstruction in the neonate. This demonstrates fluid levels in the dilated loops of gut. The distribution of air within the intestine is also important, since normally this reaches the large gut within the first few hours of life. Absence of air as shown here below the obstruction is obvious, indicating the small bowel nature of the obstruction.

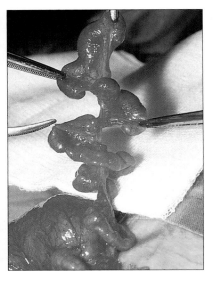

24.2   Ileal atresia. Although surgical treatment is urgent, disturbances in electrolyte balance should be corrected initially by intravenous therapy. During this period, the stomach must be kept empty by repeated gastric aspiration, continuing during transportation. Careful laparotomy is essential as atretic segments are commonly multiple (as shown) with a characteristic **'apple peel'** appearance. This anomaly is seldom associated with other malformations except in the case of duodenal atresia, which may be associated with Down's syndrome.

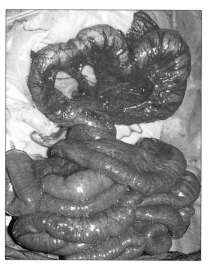

24.3 Small bowel malrotation and volvulus. If the gut fails to rotate normally during development, intestinal obstruction can occur in two ways. The caecum, whilst remaining on the left side, carries peritoneal bands from its normal site which pass across and may obstruct the duodenum. Secondly, the mesentery is attached by a narrow base, so that the chance of volvulus of the small intestine is much greater than with a normally attached mesentery (as shown). The pre-operative diagnosis was confirmed by an upper gastro–intestinal contrast study which showed the D–J flexure to the right of the mid-line.

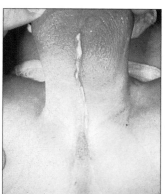

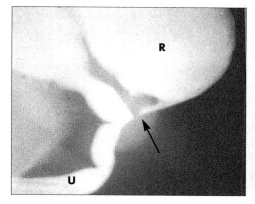

24.4 Imperforate anus and recto–urethral fistula. No anus is visible, but there is a pearly white line extending upwards towards the scrotum: this is usually consistent with a subcutaneous fistula (**left**). This should be diagnosed as soon as the baby is born, since inspection of all orifices is an integral part of the neonatal examination. If there is any external evidence of the anus, such as the dimple in this neonate, the rectum (R) probably ends low down and surgery should be able to achieve continence. Confirmation of the diagnosis is a pronogram radiograph, taken with the child upside down and a small radio opaque marker positioned on the site of the anus. This neonate has a recto–urethral fistula (**right**). U = urethra.

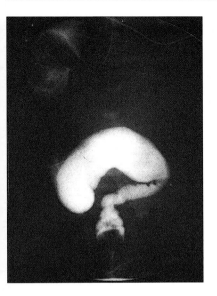

24.5 Hirschsprung's disease. This is the most common cause of intestinal obstruction in the newborn and affects boys more commonly than girls. It is due to congenital absence of the parasympathetic nerve supply and affects a variable length of the large bowel. The passage of the first meconium stool is delayed, to be passed within the first 24 hours in 10% of normal babies. Barium enema confirms the diagnosis as barium enters the narrow bowel and then passes into the dilated portion through the funnel-shaped connection. Rectal biopsy, which must include mucosa and submucosa, establishes an unequivocal diagnosis by demonstrating the absence of ganglion cells and hypertrophy of nerve fibres.

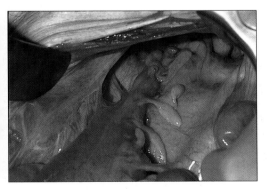

24.6 Neuronal intestinal dysplasia. The markedly dilated proximal colon narrows suddenly as it continues as the upper rectum. Histological examination of this segment in the resected specimen indicated nerve trunk hypertrophy and hyperganglionosis within the mesenteric plexus. No aganglionic segment was identified and this differentiates it from the rare but possible presentation of adult-type Hirschsprung's disease.

181

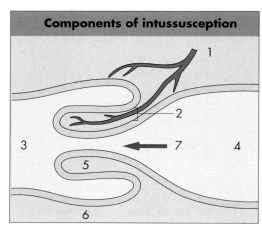

Components of intussusception

1 Blood supply
2 Mesentry
3 Distal bowel
4 Proximal bowel
5 Intussusceptum
6 Intussuscipiens
7 Direction of peristalsis

24.7 Diagram of intussusception. The bowel is invaginated in the adjacent bowel segment. The most common variant is ileo–ileal intussusception which can extend through the ileocaecal valve, although there are ileocaecal and colo–colic variants. It occurs particularly in infants between the ages of 3 and 12 months with a recent history of respiratory or gastrointestinal infection. Enlargement of Peyer's patches of lymphoid tissue, polyps or Meckel's diverticulum may form the apex of the intussusception or, in the elderly population, tumours of the small or large bowel.

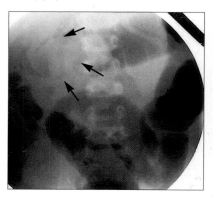
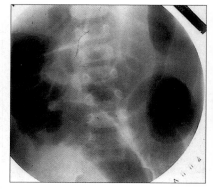

24.8 Ileal–colic intussusception. The **differential diagnosis** includes gastro–enteritis, anaphylactoid purpura, acute otitis media and acute pyelonephritis. The diagnosis is confirmed by ultrasound and an air enema (**left**) which can successfully reduce intussusceptions in approximately 70% of infants (**right**). Failure to fully reduce an intussusception is an indication for urgent surgery.

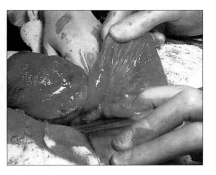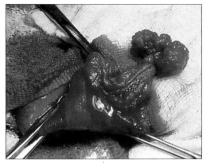

24.9 Juvenile polyp. In this child presenting with intermittent severe colicky abdominal pain, laparotomy revealed intestinal obstruction and a mass (**left**), the cause of which was a polyp at the apex of an intussusception (**right**). The small bowel was ischaemic and resection was undertaken.

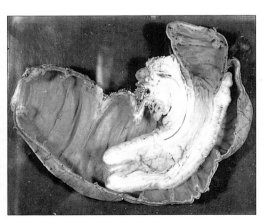

24.10 Ileal–colic intussusception. A lymphoma of the terminal ileum has intussuscepted through the ileocaecal valve into the caecal lumen. A right hemicolectomy was performed.

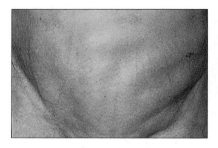
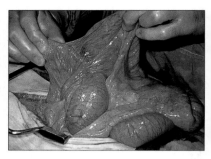

24.11 Adhesive intestinal obstruction. The most common cause of intestinal obstruction over all age groups is adhesions secondary to previous surgery. Approximately 1 in 5 patients in whom the peritoneum is breached for whatever reason will develop an episode of intestinal obstruction some time during their lifetime. The diagnosis is made on the basis of history, examination and abdominal radiography. Visible peristalsis is obvious on inspection of the abdomen (***left***). Matted small bowel adhesions were responsible in a patient with a previous perforated duodenal ulcer (***right***).

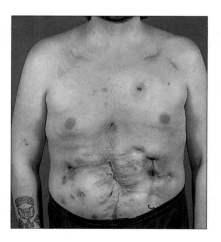

24.12 Multiple laparotomies. This patient had undergone previous gastric, gallbladder and pancreatic surgery and presented with recurrent attacks of small bowel colic, the pain based around the umbilicus. Two previous laparotomies had been performed for division of adhesions (adhesiolysis).

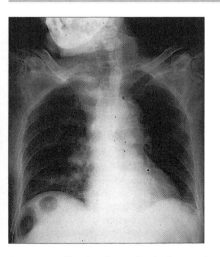
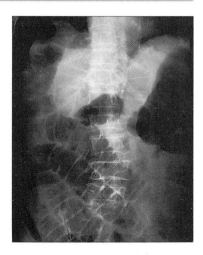

24.13 Adhesive intestinal obstruction. Loops of small bowel were unusually seen under the right hemidiaphragm on the chest radiograph (*left*). A subphrenic band adhesion between liver and diaphragm had caused an acute small bowel obstruction, 20 years after an appendicectomy (*right*).

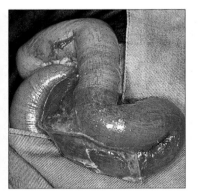
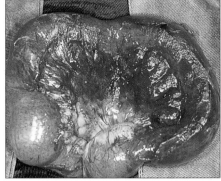

24.14 Strangulated small bowel obstruction. The development of localising tenderness was suggestive of small bowel ischaemia in the preceding patient. At laparotomy, the band adhesion was divided, the ischaemic bowel loop was released (*left*) but resection was unnecessary as the bowel was viable (*right*).

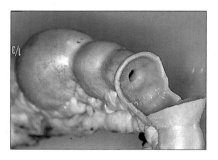

24.15 NSAID-induced small bowel diaphragms. This is a rare complication of long-term NSAID usage. The presenting features are those of intermittent small bowel obstruction. Treatment is directed at resecting the involved segment. This pathological specimen demonstrates a stenosis within the small bowel causing intestinal obstruction. This was resected and a primary anastomosis was carried out.

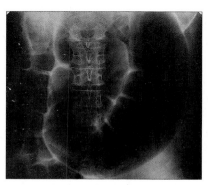

24.16 Sigmoid volvulus. This affects elderly, constipated patients, and is four times more frequent in men than in women. It is relatively rare in the UK (comprising about 2% of intestinal obstructions) but is more common in Russia, Scandinavia and Africa. The colonic loop usually twists anti-clockwise for one-half to three turns. The plain abdominal radiograph shows an enormously dilated, C-shaped, gas filled loop of sigmoid colon (**top**). A sigmoid colectomy was carried out for a grossly distended sigmoid loop (**bottom**) which failed to respond to sigmoidoscopic decompression and passage of a rectal tube.

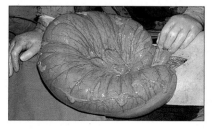

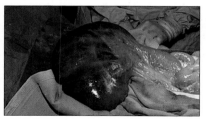

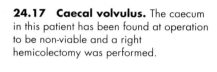

24.17 Caecal volvulus. The caecum in this patient has been found at operation to be non-viable and a right hemicolectomy was performed.

25.

SMALL BOWEL AND APPENDIX

The small intestine may become symptomatic when it **obstructs**, **bleeds**, **perforates** or has its **blood supply compromised**.

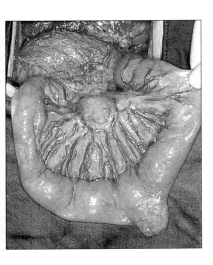

25.1 Jejunal diverticulum. This is a false diverticulum, as it does not contain all layers of the bowel wall. The diverticulum is a wide-mouthed sac caused by herniation of the mucosa on the mesenteric border. As in the sigmoid colon, complications include bleeding, inflammation, perforation or, if multiple, malabsorption due to accumulation of intestinal organisms within the diverticula.

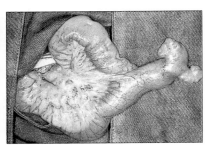

25.2 Meckel's diverticulum. This is the most common congenital abnormality of the gastro–intestinal tract (present in about 2% of the population) and results from persistence of the vitello–intestinal duct. It is a true diverticulum containing all layers, and arises from the antemesenteric border of the ileum, 60–70 cm from the ileo–caecal valve, and is on average 5 cm long (range 1–15 cm).

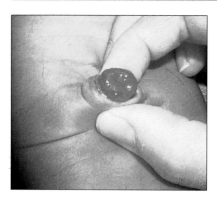

25.3 Umbilical fistula. In 5% of patients with Meckel's diverticulum, a fibrous cord (the remaining portion of the vitello–intestinal duct) connects it to the umbilicus. Infrequently, the small bowel may fistulate through the Meckel's diverticulum into the umbilicus. The principal **differential diagnosis** is that of a patent urachus to the urinary bladder.

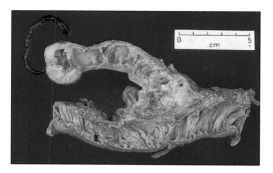

25.4 Symptomatic Meckel's diverticulum. Only 5% of Meckel's diverticula cause symptoms. Heterotrophic tissue, particularly gastric mucosa, is frequently found in 50% of symptomatic diverticula. An acute ulcer causing pain and occult GI blood loss was responsible for this patient's symptoms. Technetium[99] scintiscanning uptake with cimetidine enhancement localised heterotrophic gastric mucosa. A 6-week course of cimetidine cured the patient's symptoms and elective surgery removed the offending Meckel's diverticulum. On sectioning, there was no evidence of acute ulceration, but histology confirmed ectopic gastric mucosa.

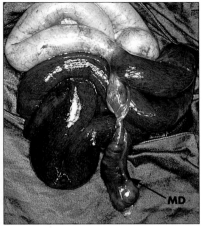

25.5 Internal hernia caused by a Meckel's diverticulum. This patient presented with severe colicky periumbilical pain and vomiting. The 14 cm long Meckel's diverticulum (MD) was attached by a congenital band to the ileo–caecal angle, around which the terminal three feet of small bowel had herniated. The non-viable bowel was resected.

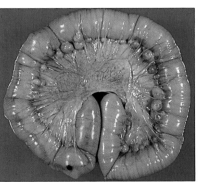

25.6 Multiple ileal diverticulosis.
The ileum is less frequently affected by multiple diverticula compared to the jejunum, and their presence may be an incidental finding at surgery or on presentation with one of the complications associated with diverticulosis.

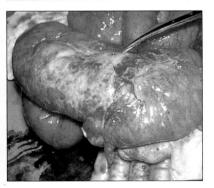

25.7 Perforated terminal ileitis.
Crohn's disease may present in a similar manner to that of acute appendicitis. A 22-year-old male had a history of several bouts of episodic diarrhoea associated with recurrent abdominal pain, lassitude and pyrexia. Although the terminal ileum has perforated in this patient, a much more common presentation is that of simple terminal ileitis. Consider a **differential diagnosis** of eosinophilic ileitis, other inflammatory bowel disease or lymphoma.

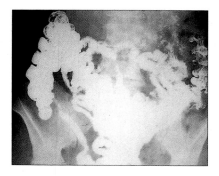

25.8 Crohn's disease. A small bowel enema was performed electively which shows thickening of the small bowel, narrowing of the lumen and separation of bowel loops which coincide with evidence of tissue destruction and ulceration, spike-like fissures and a 'cobblestone' appearance of the mucosa. Should the enema give an equivocal diagnosis, a full thickness small bowel biopsy may be required.

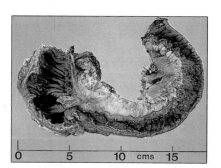

25.9 Crohn's disease of the distal ileum. This open pathological specimen shows a typical 'cobblestone' mucosa with deep ulcers present. Although the small bowel enema suggested the diseased segment was in the jejunum, on-table enteroscopy demonstrated that the proximal small bowel was clear and that the distal small bowel was diseased. Where strictures are short, multiple stricturoplasties may be undertaken, thus preserving small bowel length.

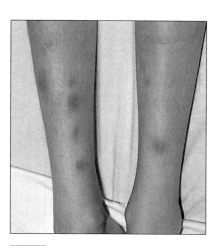

25.10 Erythema nodosum. In addition to the aphthous ulcers in his mouth, this 14-year-old boy had these painful tender lesions on both legs which are characteristic of erythema nodosum. Together with his presentation of acute abdominal pain, a presumptive diagnosis of acute Crohn's disease was made. This was subsequently confirmed by barium follow through examination although he did not require surgery.

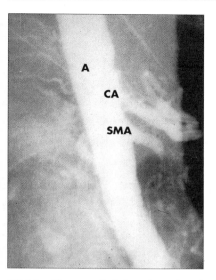 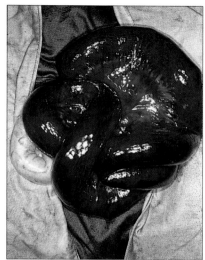

25.11 Mesenteric infarction. Thrombotic or embolic occlusion of the superior mesenteric artery is an acute abdominal emergency. In most patients, the thrombosis is the final event in widespread arteriopathy. Emboli, usually originating from intra-cardiac thrombus in patients with atrial fibrillation or recent myocardial infarction, account for occlusion in one-third of cases, as shown in this superior mesenteric angiogram (*left*). A=aorta; CA=coeliac axis; SMA=superior mesenteric artery. A high index of suspicion is required because, unless the presentation and diagnosis are made quickly, the condition is uniformly fatal with massive mesenteric infarction (*right*).

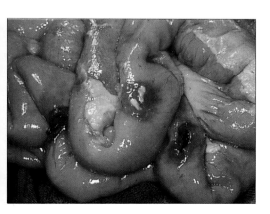

25.12 Polyarteritis nodosa of the small bowel. The multiple perforations shown here at operation occurred throughout the length of the small bowel and are surrounded by erythematous serosal areas. The principal **differential diagnosis** of multiple perforations includes typhoid, uraemia, potassium ingestion and non-steroidal anti-inflammatory drug ingestion.

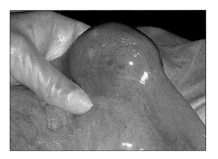 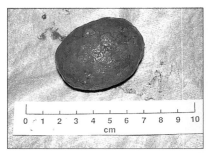

25.13 Gallstone ileus. This 75-year-old presented with an acute small bowel obstruction in a virgin abdomen (**left**). A large gallstone had impacted in the distal ileum causing the obstruction and was removed by proximal displacement and enterotomy (**right**). The gallbladder is usually left undisturbed to avoid unnecessary and hazardous cholecystectomy. The diagnosis of gallstone ileus can be made pre-operatively on the abdominal radiograph which shows the presence of a small bowel obstruction and gas within the biliary tree.

SMALL BOWEL NEOPLASMS

Classification of Small Bowel Neoplasms
Small bowel neoplasms are rare, comprising less than 5 per cent of all gastro-intestinal malignancies. Benign lesions are ten times as common as malignant lesions. Small bowel tumours may present with **intestinal bleeding, obstruction, intussusception** or a **volvulus**.

Benign
- Adenoma.
- Leiomyoma.
- Lipoma.
- Multiple polyposis (Peutz–Jeuger syndrome).

Malignant
- Adenocarcinoma.
- Carcinoid.
- Lymphoma.
- Leiomyosarcoma.
- Secondary invasion (from stomach, colon, bladder, ovary).

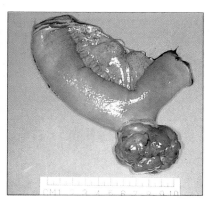
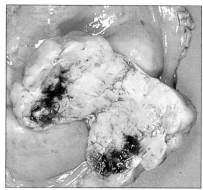

25.14 Leiomyoma. Occult blood loss caused a sustained microcytic anaemia. Laparotomy found a Meckel's-like lesion in the ileum (***left***) but it had a suspicious macroscopic appearance. The lesion was solid, with an area of haemorrhage (***right***). Histology confirmed a benign smooth muscle tumour.

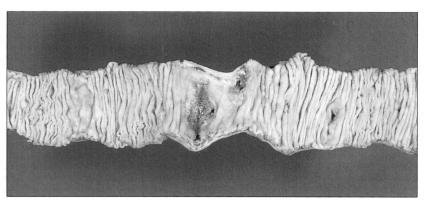

25.15 Small bowel lymphoma. This pathological specimen shows multiple lymphomatous nodules in the terminal ileum. This pathology may present with free perforation causing peritonitis. Any unresected lymphomatous deposits may perforate as they respond to chemotherapy.

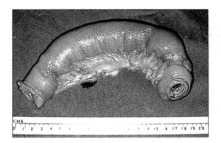 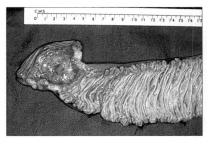

25.16 Small bowel carcinoma. These are rare tumours and presentation is normally as a small bowel obstruction (**left**). Initially the stricture was thought to be benign but, on opening the bowel, there was an obvious, ulcerating fibrotic lesion (**right**).

APPENDIX

The **appendix** is a true diverticulum arising from the dependent pole of the caecum. It can be identified at surgery by the convergence of the taeni coli on the root of the appendix. The most common position is retrocaecal (65 per cent of patients). In 20 per cent the appendix is located in the pelvic region and in the remaining 15 per cent of patients it is either subcaecal, paracaecal, pre- or post-ileal. Knowledge of these variations is important as its presentation is dependent upon the position of this appendage.

Acute appendicitis is predominantly a disease of Western civilisation and is uncommon in Africa and Asia. Acute appendicitis remains the most common abdominal surgical emergency in childhood, adolescence and early life. Less than 2 per cent of cases occur in infants under two years of age, and the incidence is highest during the second and the third decades of life. Thereafter it declines, and less than 5 per cent of cases occur in patients over 60 years.

Mortality associated with appendicitis is rare but, if there is a delay in presentation or diagnosis, **complications of appendicitis**, including gangrene, necrosis, perforation, abscess formation, septicaemia and portal vein thrombosis, can result in substantial morbidity.

An **appendix mass** may develop when presentation has been delayed. It is formed by omentum and small bowel being wrapped around the inflamed appendix. Clinically there is a low grade pyrexia, elevated white cell count, and a right iliac fossa mass. The diagnosis may be confirmed by ultrasound. Most respond to antibiotic therapy but should an abscess develop, then drainage is required.

Differential Diagnosis of Acute Appendicitis

The following conditions should be considered in the **differential diagnosis**:

- Mesenteric adenitis.
- Urinary tract infection.
- Gynaecological pathology (ectopic pregnancy and ruptured ovarian cysts, pelvic inflammatory disease, ovarian torsion).
- Crohn's disease.
- *Yersinia* ileitis.
- Meckel's diverticulitis.
- Caecal carcinoma.
- Psoas abscess.

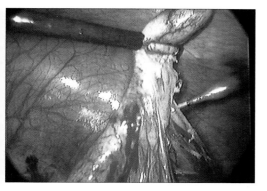

25.17 Acute appendicitis at laparoscopy. This 15-year-old girl presented with a 24-hour history of central colicky abdominal pain associated with nausea, vomiting and loss of appetite, which then moved to the right iliac fossa and became much more localised. There was associated tachycardia, pyrexia, localised tenderness, guarding and rebound. After a short period of observation, she was subjected to laparoscopy and an acutely inflamed appendix was identified and removed laparoscopically. The patient went home the following day with appropriate antibiotic cover.

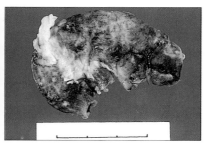

25.18 Gangrenous appendicitis. This perforated necrotic specimen occurred in a 27-year-old man who had a one-week history of lower abdominal pain. He had chosen to ignore his right iliac fossa pain before collapsing and presenting with septic shock. Following emergency appendicectomy, he developed adult respiratory distress syndrome from which he recovered.

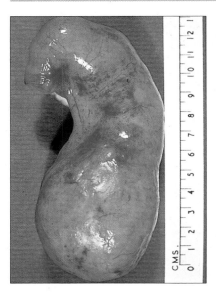 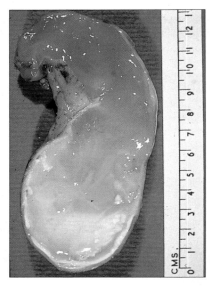

25.19 Mucocele of the appendix. One of the possible consequences of conservatively treating suspected appendicitis is the development of a mucocele (**left**). It is advisable to remove such lesions as there is the risk of pseudomyxoma peritonei if rupture occurs and mucus contents spill into the peritoneal cavity (**right**).

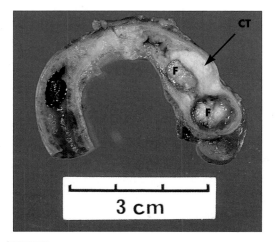

25.20 Appendiceal carcinoid. The appendix is the most common site of GI carcinoid tumours (CT), followed by the small bowel. It is often an incidental finding following appendicectomy. The opened pathological specimen shows the appendiceal tumour, with faecoliths (F), in the lumen of the appendix. Such tumours rarely metastasise to the liver unless they arise from the small intestine.

26.

COLON

The large bowel and rectum are derived embryologically from the distal midgut, the entire hindgut and portions of the cloaca. The colon begins at the ileocaecal valve with the caecum in the right iliac fossa, extends upwards as the ascending colon to the hepatic flexure, then across as the transverse colon up to the splenic flexure, descending towards the pelvis as the descending colon and continuing as the sigmoid loop. At the pelvic brim, the recto–sigmoid junction is formed with the upper third of the rectum being above the peritoneal reflection and the lower two-thirds below the pelvic peritoneum, running towards the anus. The last 4 cm comprise the anal canal.

The **cardinal symptoms and signs** of colonic disease are: abdominal pain; alteration in bowel habit; the passage of blood or mucus per rectum; mass; abdominal distension and hepatomegaly. Weight loss, malaise and anaemia are important non-specific features. **Risk factors** for colorectal cancer are family history, country of origin, slow intestinal transit, longstanding inflammatory bowel disease, adenomatous polyps, familial adenomatous polyposis and villous adenomata.

Diagnosis

- General examination.
- Abdominal and digital rectal examination.
- Faecal occult blood testing.
- Full blood count and liver function tests.
- Carcinoembryonic antigen (CEA).*
- Sigmoidoscopy.
- Colonoscopy.
- Plain abdominal radiography.
- Double contrast barium enema.
- Ultrasonography of liver and kidneys.*
- Intra-operative ultrasonography.*
- CT scanning.*

* if carcinoma suspected

Lymphatic Drainage of the Large Bowl

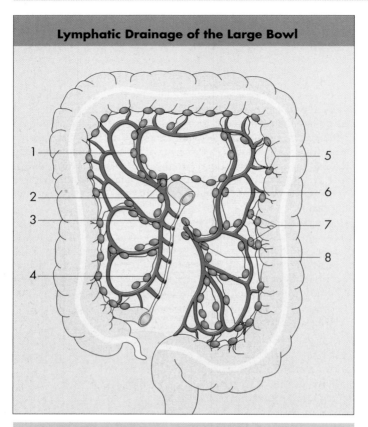

1 Middle colic nodes	5 Epicolic nodes
2 Superior mesenteric nodes	6 Left colic nodes
3 Right colic nodes	7 Paracolic nodes
4 Ileo–colic nodes	8 Inferior mesenteric nodes

26.1 Lymphatic drainage of the large bowel. Lymph drains in the colon to epicolic nodes on the bowel wall and then to paracolic nodes between the marginal artery and the bowel. Lymph then drains from the intermediate nodes on the main vessels to two principal nodes alongside the origin of the superior and inferior mesenteric vessels. Lymph from the rectum drains upwards to superior rectal and inferior mesenteric nodes, or laterally along the middle rectal vessels to the internal ileac nodes. Drainage of the anal canal and perianal skin is to the inguinal nodes.

DIVERTICULAR DISEASE

Diverticula of the large bowel are rare under the age of 35 years. By 65 years of age, at least 30 per cent of the general population are affected. These are false diverticulae of the pulsion type which emerge between the mesenteric and ante-mesenteric taenia at the sites of penetration of small blood vessels.

Inflammation of diverticula (**diverticulitis**), particularly in the sigmoid colon, may cause severe, localising, left iliac fossa pain and a palpable tender mass. If this fails to settle with antibiotic therapy (metronidazole and cephalosporin), laparotomy with resection of the inflamed colon may be necessary. The principal options are a Hartmann's procedure (terminal colostomy with oversewing of the rectal stump), or alternatively a left hemicolectomy with primary anastomosis.

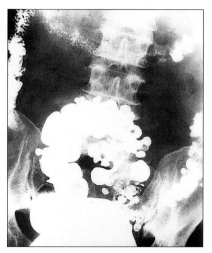 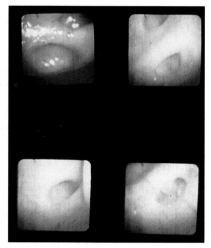

26.2 Diverticulosis. This contrast study shows extensive diverticular disease in the sigmoid colon (***left***). This 67-year-old woman complained of lower abdominal and left iliac fossa pain, alteration in bowel habit and intermittent rectal bleeding. To exclude a neoplastic cause for her bleeding, flexible sigmoidoscopy confirmed multiple diverticula (***right***). Endoscopic examination can be difficult because of circular muscle spasm which gives rise to the pain associated with diverticular disease. Her symptoms improved on a high fibre diet and anti-spasmodics. Diverticula can become inflamed, bleed, perforate or a segment of affected bowel may fibrose and stricture.

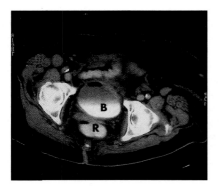

26.3 Colo–vesical fistula. This 80-year-old woman presented with pneumaturia and altered bowel habit. Flexible sigmoidoscopy demonstrated a stricturing lesion at 12 cm and biopsy was normal. The abdominal CT scan shows gas within the bladder (B), indicative of a colo–vesical fistula. There was an associated 7 cm mass in the recto–sigmoid (R). Other causes of colo–vesical fistula are Crohn's disease, carcinoma and radiation enteritis. Treatment was by anterior resection of the rectum and repair of the bladder.

ULCERATIVE COLITIS

Ulcerative colitis, the aetiology of which is unknown, has an incidence of 5 new cases per 100,000 population per year. It most commonly affects young adults, particularly women, in a male to female ratio of 1:1.5. Although it is more common in first degree relatives, 90 per cent of patients have no family history. It is primarily a disease of the large bowel although systemic manifestations similar to those of Crohn's disease are described. These often disappear completely when all the affected bowel has been removed.

Complications of ulcerative colitis include: carcinoma; delay in sexual development; malnutrition; anaemia; ano–rectal complications; benign strictures; pseudopolyp formation; and **systemic complications** such as erythema nodosum, pyoderma gangrenosum, iritis, hepatitis, sclerosing cholangitis and ankylosing spondylitis.

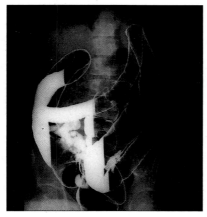

26.4 Ulcerative colitis. The barium enema shows the characteristic loss of haustrations, reduction in the calibre of the bowel, pseudopolyp formation and a fluffy outline of the mucosa. Included in the **differential diagnosis** is *amoebic* colitis, Crohn's disease and, in the elderly, ischaemic colitis.

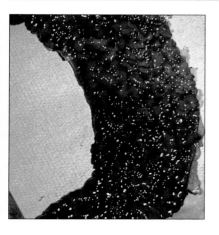

26.5 Toxic megacolon. This patient, with a 3-year history of ulcerative colitis, presented with an exacerbation associated with passing large and frequent quantities of blood and mucus from the rectum, pyrexia, abdominal pain and tenderness. Plain abdominal radiography showed the characteristic features of toxic megacolon which is at risk of perforation and causing septicaemic shock. There was no dramatic response to high dose steroids and antibiotics, and emergency colectomy was necessary (specimen shown).

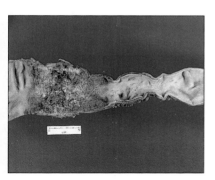

26.6 Pathological specimen of longstanding ulcerative colitis. This panproctocolectomy specimen was removed from a 42-year-old man with a 15-year history of ulcerative colitis which had run an intermittent course. At annual colonoscopy, sequential colonic biopsies demonstrated areas of marked dysplasia proximal to an obvious cancer in the transverse colon. Carcinomas arising in colitic colons tend to pursue a much more aggressive course.

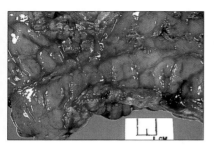

26.7 Crohn's disease. Crohn's disease differs from ulcerative colitis in its histological features, and macroscopically there are 'skip' lesions with 'cobblestone' mucosa, whereas disease in ulcerative colitis usually is continuous from the rectum and extends stepwise into the proximal colon.

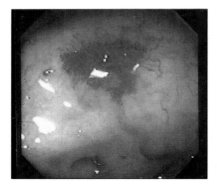

26.8 Angiodysplasia. This colonoscopic view demonstrates an angiodysplastic lesion in the right colon in an elderly patient who presented with massive rectal bleeding and shock. The **differential diagnosis** includes carcinoma and diverticular disease. If bleeding is not severe, colonoscopy may be helpful in establishing the cause, but continuing severe haemorrhage is an indication for surgery. In this frail patient, the lesion was dealt with by heater probe coagulation.

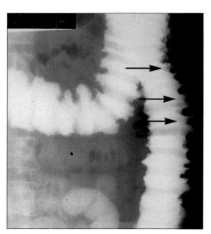

26.9 Ischaemic colitis. Single contrast enema shows 'thumb-printing' of the colonic mucosa in the region of the splenic flexure, due to oedema of the mucosa and confirmed by a limited barium enema. The most precarious blood supply to the large bowel is at the splenic flexure which, in this patient, was compromised by sustained hypotension following a massive bleed from a gastric ulcer.

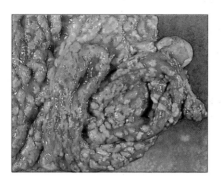

26.10 Pathological appearance of pseudomembranous colitis. This condition is associated with the use of antibiotics. There is necrosis of the mucous membrane of the colon, associated with profuse watery diarrhoea, toxaemia, shock and collapse. The diagnosis is confirmed by biopsy and isolation of *Clostridium difficile* toxin in the stool or in the pseudomembrane. Treatment consists of intravenous fluid replacement and vancomycin or metronidazole.

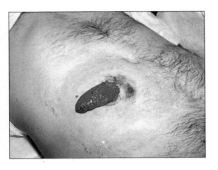

26.11 Ileostomy. These are usually sited in the left iliac fossa and differ from colostomies in that a spout is formed in order to minimise the irritant effect of small bowel content on the surrounding skin. In this Crohn's patient, a peristomal fistula has developed, as well as prolapse of the ileostomy spout.

COLORECTAL NEOPLASMS

Classification of Colorectal Neoplasms

Benign
- Metaplastic polyp.
- Adenomatous/villous polyps.
- Familial adenomatous polyposis.
- Leiomyoma.

Malignant
- Adenocarcinoma.
- Squamous cell carcinoma.
- Carcinoid.
- Lymphoma.
- Leiomyosarcoma.
- Secondary invasion (from stomach, colon, bladder, ovary).

Carcinoma of the **colon and rectum** is second only to lung cancer as a cause of death from cancer in the Western society. Scotland has the highest incidence of colorectal cancer in the world. With 39 new cases per 100,000 population, and 1800 deaths each year. It is predominantly a disease of older people and is uncommon before the age of 40. Overall, males and females have an equal incidence, but there is a distinct difference in distribution: cancer of the rectum is more common in males and cancer of the caecum is more common in females.

Distribution
Two-thirds of large bowel cancers originate in the rectum and the sigmoid colon. A further 10 per cent occur in the caecum, and the remainder are distributed through the rest of the large bowel. In 4 per cent of patients, at the time of presentation, synchronous tumours may be present, while in 1 per cent a metachronous tumour will develop in the colon during follow-up within 3 years.

Stages of Colorectal Cancer (modified Dukes' classification)

Stage	*Definition*
A	Growth confined to bowel wall.
B	Spread through the bowel wall.
C	Involvement of regional lymph nodes.

C_1: Few nodes involved near the primary growth, but some nodes in the chain are free from metastases below the ligature on main regional vessels.

C_2: Continuous chain of nodes containing metastases right up to the ligature on the main regional vessels.

D	Distant metastases.

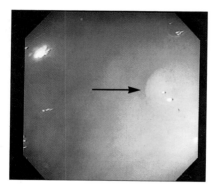

26.12 Metaplastic polyp. These are very common, usually small and easily removed by biopsy forceps. They may be multiple and need to be differentiated from adenomatous and villous polyps.

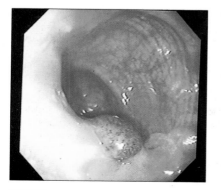

26.13 Adenomatous polyp. This is a true neoplasm, and accounts for 90% of neoplastic polyps of the colon. They are most commonly pedunculated, as shown here, and a careful search is required to identify others. This lesion was removed by colonic polypectomy. In one-third of cases, polyps are multiple with their distribution similar to that of carcinoma.

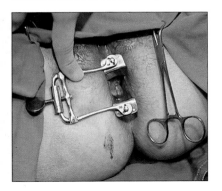

26.14 Villous adenoma. This tumour accounts for 10% of neoplastic polyps of the large bowel and is most commonly found in the rectum and sigmoid colon. Because of the extensive mucus secretion, patients may present with mucous discharge but, if the lesion is large, dehydration, hypokalaemia, weakness and metabolic alkalosis may result. Rectal bleeding is a late sign and is suggestive of malignant change. In this patient the polyp prolapsed through the anus.

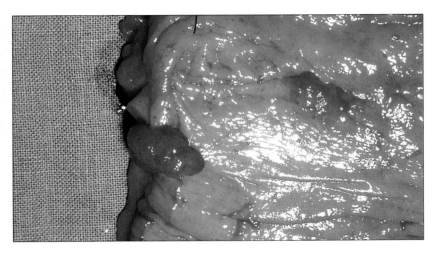

26.15 Familial adenomatous polyposis. This is a rare hereditary disease transmitted by an autosomal-dominant gene. Sessile and pedunculated adenomas develop during late childhood in the large bowel, ranging in number from several to many hundreds of adenomas, and in this pathological specimen approximately 40. The rectum is almost always involved and presentation in unscreened individuals is heralded by rectal bleeding, diarrhoea and mucous discharge. Although malignant change is inevitable in individuals who develop polyposis, histology of these polyps showed moderate dysplasia only. Total colectomy and ileo–rectal anastomosis was carried out in this 28-year-old male. Rectal polyps require regular surveillance and biopsy to detect malignant change.

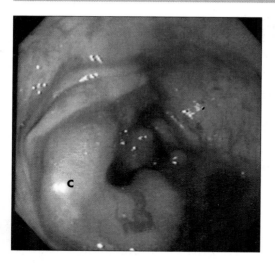

26.16 Colonoscopic appearance of an ulcerative tumour. This carcinoma (C) was diagnosed at the caecal pole in a patient presenting with melaena and weight loss. Treatment consisted of right hemicolectomy and, although there was no evidence of hepatic spread, the lymph nodes were involved with metastatic disease, indicating that this was a Dukes' C tumour.

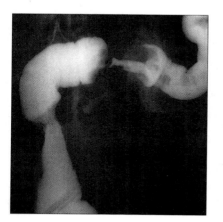

26.17 Large bowel carcinoma. The barium enema shows the typical shouldering 'apple-core' appearance of a carcinoma.

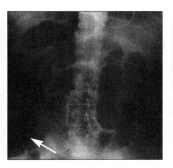
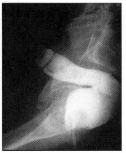
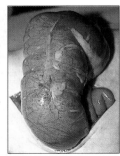

26.18 Obstructing carcinoma of the recto–sigmoid junction. The abdominal radiograph shows marked caecal distension and small bowel dilatation (***left***). An urgent gastrograffin enema shows clear cut-off at the recto–sigmoid junction indicative of an obstructing carcinoma (***middle***). Massive caecal dilatation (***right***) with serosal splitting necessitated emergency total colectomy and ileo–rectal anastomosis. Alternatively, the rectum could have been cross-stapled and an ileostomy formed where there is any doubt regarding the bowel viability at the anastomosis.

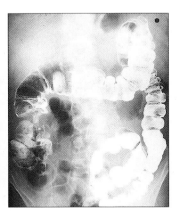
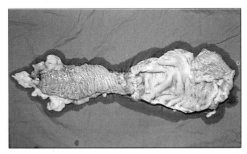

26.19 Carcinoma of the ascending colon. Barium enema, carried out for investigation of melaena, shows a stricturing lesion in the right colon (***left***). This was an annular tumour which was resected and a primary anastomosis was carried out (***right***). Subsequent histological examination confirmed involvement through the entire thickness of the bowel wall and of adjacent lymph nodes (Dukes' stage C).

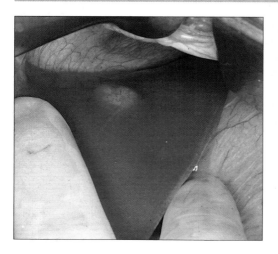

26.20 Hepatic metastases. A large sigmoid tumour has metastasised to the liver, staging this cancer as Dukes' D. Isolated metastases may be amenable to resection after full staging investigations.

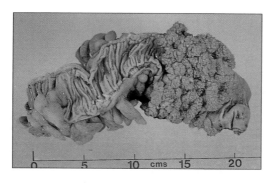

26.21 Polypoidal carcinoma of the colon. This is one of the three variants of large bowel cancer, the other two being stenosing and ulcerating lesions. Polypoidal lesions can bleed, intussuscept or cause intestinal obstruction.

27.

ANAL CANAL AND RECTUM

Anatomy of the Anal Canal

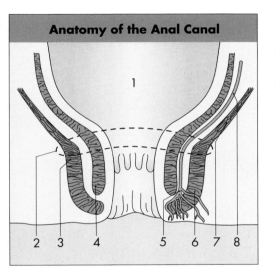

1 Rectum
2 Anorectal ring
3 Puborectalis
4 Internal sphincter
5 Longitudinal intersphincteric muscle
6 External sphincter
7 Levator ani
8 Longitudinal muscle of rectal wall

27.1 Diagrammatic representation of the anal canal. The lower border of the puborectalis is in continuity with the external sphincter (both striated muscles and thus under voluntary control). The anorectal ring is the condensed ring of muscle formed by the puborectalis and the upper edges of the internal and external sphincters. This ring can be felt rectally and is vital to continence. The dentate line, 2.5 cm from the anal verge, corresponds to the line of fusion between the endoderm of the hindgut and the ectoderm of the anal pit. The canal above this line is innervated by the autonomic nervous system whereas, beneath the dentate line, it is lined by modified skin innervated by the peripheral nervous system. Histologically, there is a gradual transition from mucus-secreting columnar mucosa to stratified squamous epithelium. Continence is maintained by a combination of both internal and external sphincter tones.

Differential Diagnosis of Pruritus Ani

Anorectal disease
- Haemorrhoids.
- Fissure.
- Fistula.
- Proctitis.
- Polyps.

Skin disease
- Psoriasis.
- Lichen planus.
- Contact eczema.
- Pre-malignant keratosis.

Infection
- Candidiasis.
- Other fungal infections.
- Threadworm.
- Viral papillomata.

Miscellaneous
- Drug reaction (quinidine, colchicine).
- Obesity.

Differential Diagnosis of Severe Anal Pain

The principal differential diagnoses are **prolapsed haemorrhoids** and **perianal haematoma**, the latter of which presents with sudden onset of severe anal pain, with the development of a submucosal haematoma following a rupture of a perianal vein. This is exquisitely tender and managed by simple incision and evacuation of the haematoma under local anaesthesia with immediate relief of symptoms. An **anal fissure** causes severe burning pain on defaecation which may persist for several hours, minor bleeding, excoriation and pruritus. The pain may be so intense that defaecation is avoided. Fissures are usually anterior or posterior, and a tear extends from the anal verge to the dentate line in the posterior midline. Treatment is by conservative measures with local anaesthetic ointments, suppositories and, if this fails, by lateral subcutaneous internal sphincterotomy.

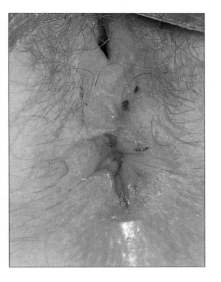

27.2 Excoriation associated with pruritus ani. This is a common condition which occurs more frequently in men, especially between the ages of 30 and 60 years. Causal factors can only be identified in approximately 50% of patients. This patient with mild excoriation had a posterior anal fissure.

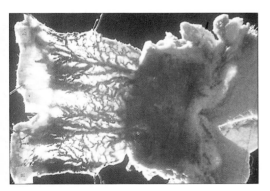 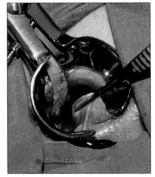

27.3 Haemorrhoids. Haemorrhoids remain one of the most common ailments of Western society, although their aetiology remains uncertain (**left**). They commonly develop or increase in size during pregnancy and are associated with constipation and straining at stool. The haemorrhoidal cushions lie in the left lateral, right anterior and right posterior positions relative to the anal canal. Small accessory piles are often present between the three vein masses. Rectal bleeding is the usual presentation and treatment is either by submucosal sclerosant injection, rubber banding or infra-red coagulation. More extensive haemorrhoids or those failing to respond to these interventions, may require surgical excision as demonstrated (**right**).
(Left) by courtesy of Thomson, WH in *Oxford Textbook of Surgery*, vol 1 (1994).

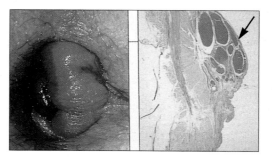

27.4 Prolapsed thrombosed haemorrhoids. This is an exceedingly painful condition which can be managed conservatively with bed rest, ice packs and topical anaesthesia, or alternatively by emergency haemorrhoidectomy with instant relief of pain (*left*). Histology (*right*) shows the thrombosis.

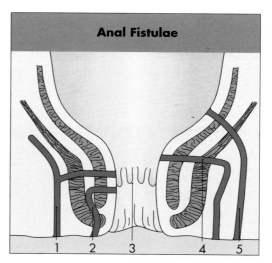

Anal Fistulae

1 Ischiorectal
2 Low anal
3 Anus
4 High anal
5 Pelvirectal

27.5 Diagrammatic representation of sites of anal fistulae. These may be simple or complex. Definition of the fistulous tract by fistulogram or MRI scanning is imperative, as this will determine the surgical approach. **Goodsall's rule** holds that a fistula with an external opening in the front of a transverse line through the anus will generally open into the anal canal at the nearest point on its circumference. Fistulae with external openings behind this line tend to open internally in the posterior midline, and may extend behind the anal canal on both sides, forming a horseshoe fistula.

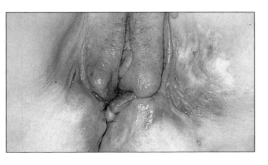

27.6 Fistula-in-ano. This patient has Crohn's disease and presented with recurrent fistulation (**top**). The fistulous tract is defined by contrast (**bottom**). 40% of patients with Crohn's disease have anal manifestations. Rectal biopsy is mandatory to exclude other conditions such as ulcerative colitis, tuberculosis, HIV infection and venereal lymphogranuloma.

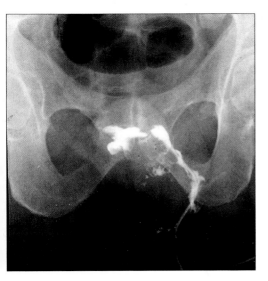

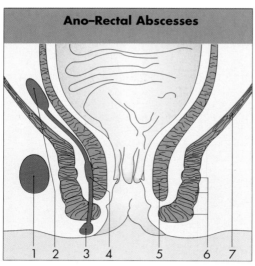

Ano–Rectal Abscesses

1 Ischiorectal abscess
2 High intermuscular abscess
3 Perianal/subcutaneous abscess
4 Intersphincteric abscess
5 Internal sphincter
6 External sphincter
7 Levator ani

27.7 Diagrammatic representation of sites of ano–rectal abscesses.
Ano–rectal abscesses are a common cause of admission to hospital. They are 2–3 times more common in males than in females, the highest incidence occurring in the 3rd and 4th decades. Most arise spontaneously but the infection may arise in the anal glands, pass into the inter-sphincteric plane and then track inferiorly to present as a peri-anal abscess, laterally to form an ischiorectal abscess, or superiorly to produce a high intersphincteric abscess.

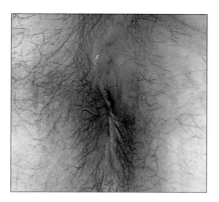

27.8 Recurrent perianal abscess.
This is common and presents as an acute, painful, tender swelling at the anal verge. Systemic upset is minimal and simple incision, drainage, curettage, irrigation and light packing, followed by daily dressing with an alginate-based dressing, is required. Where abscesses of this nature are recurrent (1–2 o'clock position), then an underlying fistula should be sought.

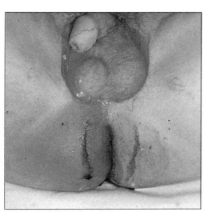

27.9 Ischiorectal abscess. This is also common and produces a brawny, diffuse induration lateral to the anus. The swelling is painful and tender but fluctuation occurs late. Systemic upset is pronounced. The swelling may be palpable on digital rectal examination and infection may extend behind the anal canal as a horseshoe abscess involving both ischiorectal fossae. Incision and drainage is the method of treatment. Primary closure of abscesses under antibiotic cover is carried out by a minority of surgeons.

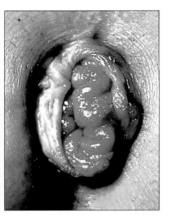

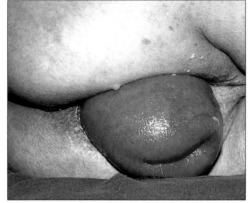

27.10 Rectal prolapse. Rectal mucosal prolapse (**left**) is a prelude to complete prolapse (**right**) where there is an intussusception of the rectum, which results in the whole thickness of the bowel protruding through the anus. Approximately 85% of affected adults are women, and older females are particularly at risk. Digital examination in this elderly woman revealed poor sphincter tone, laxity of the anus, and gross faecal incontinence. Depending on the patient's fitness, surgical treatment of complete prolapse in the frail patients can be aimed at perineal excision of the rectum and anal sphincter plication. Alternatively, there are a variety of abdominal procedures which include anterior resection and rectopexy.

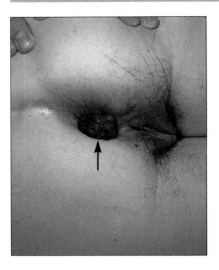

27.11 Rectal villous adenoma.
This lesion was detected in a 53-year-old female by rectal examination during a routine admission for inguinal hernia repair where the lesion had prolapsed through the anus. Proctoscopic examination and biopsy confirmed a benign tumour. Transanal submucosal resection was performed under general anaesthesia.

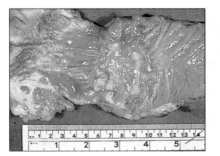

27.12 Rectal carcinoma. This 73-year-old woman presented with a 6-month history of intermittent rectal bleeding which she attributed to her piles, early morning diarrhoea, urgency, tenesmus and the feeling of incomplete evacuation of the bowel. Preservation of the anal sphincters was not possible and an abdomino–perineal excision of the rectum was undertaken.

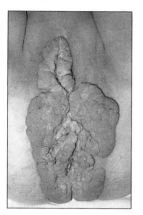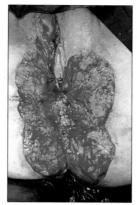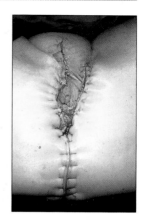

27.13 **Anal warts.** Extensive anal warts (**left**) interfered with defaecation and required radical excision (**middle**). The resultant defect was closed by mobilizing the adjacent skin flaps (**right**).

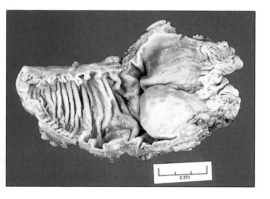

27.14 **Squamous cell carcinoma of the anus.** Smaller lesions may respond to radiotherapy but in the patient there was a progressive increase in size of the lesion, necessitating resection of rectum and anus. Lymphatic spread occurs to the groins. If groin nodes are involved, bilateral groin dissection may be undertaken.

28.

HERNIA

A hernia is a swelling caused by the protrusion of part or the whole of an organ or other tissue through a normal or abnormal defect in the wall surrounding the space in which the organ or tissue is normally situated.

Abdominal wall hernias are one of the most common causes for referral to the general surgeon. They can occur at any site, often following natural orifices in the abdominal wall through which structures enter and leave the abdominal cavity. These are the umbilicus, the inguinal, femoral and obturator canals, and the oesophageal hiatus in the diaphragm. Other hernias protrude through areas of weakness in the abdominal musculature, and these include direct inguinal hernias, incisional hernias due to previous surgery, and epigastric hernias due to defects in the fibrous layer of the linea alba.

Hernias in the groin region account for between 75 and 80 per cent of all abdominal hernias. There are **three common types: indirect inguinal** (60 per cent), **direct inguinal** (25 per cent) and **femoral** (15 per cent). The majority (85 per cent) of inguinal hernias occurs in males. Femoral hernias are more common in females, but indirect inguinal hernias are still the most common hernia in women.

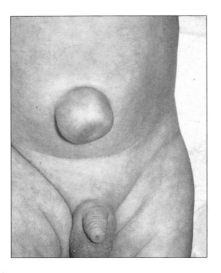

28.1 Umbilical hernia. Over all age groups, this is the most common hernia present in man. By definition, all neonates at birth must have an abdominal wall defect at the umbilicus to allow blood flow to and from the placenta. By the age of one year, 90% of the defects at the umbilicus have closed and by two years of age, 99% have closed. Surgery therefore is not indicated for umbilical hernia below the age of three years.

Anatomy of the Inguinal Canal

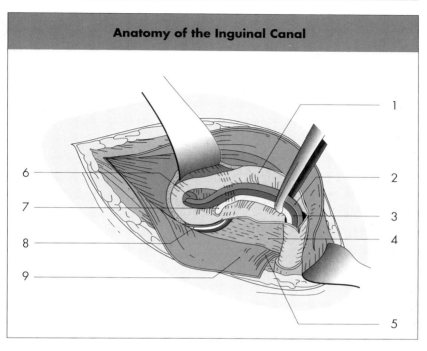

28.2 Diagrammatic representation of the inguinal canal. The inguinal canal contains the spermatic cord in males and the round ligament in females. Both these structures exit the abdominal cavity at the deep inguinal ring which lies 2 cm above the mid-inguinal point. The superficial inguinal ring lies just above and medial to the pubic tubercle. The deep inguinal ring is bounded medially by the inferior epigastric vessels. Inguinal hernias which arise lateral to the inferior epigastric vessels through the deep inguinal ring are termed **indirect inguinal** hernias. Those arising medially through the posterior wall of the inguinal canal medial to the vessels are **direct hernias**. The anterior wall of the inguinal canal is the external oblique.

1 Internal spermatic fascia
2 Spermatic veins
3 Testicular artery
4 Transversalis fascia
5 Superficial inguinal ring
6 Deep inguinal ring
7 Vas
8 Inferior epigastric vessels
9 External oblique muscle, opened

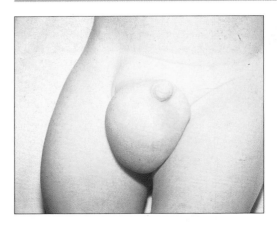
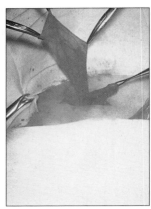

28.3 Paediatric inguinal hernia. The diagnosis is made by the appearance of an inguinal swelling (***left***), often present when the child cries or strains and confirmed by gently rubbing the two surfaces of the inguinal sac together which gives a 'silky sensation'. Boys are more commonly affected and the hernia may be associated with an undescended testicle. Herniotomy and excision of the delicate gossamer sac (***right***) are all that is required.

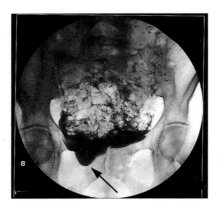

28.4 Herniogram. In adults presenting with groin pain and no obvious cough impulse or swelling, inguinal and femoral hernias may be diagnosed by a herniogram. Contrast is injected into the peritoneal cavity in a dependent manner with the patient rolled on to the side of the pain. In this patient a small, indirect inguinal hernia was found and confirmed at operation. However, in most patients, groin pain is due to musculo–skeletal disorders.

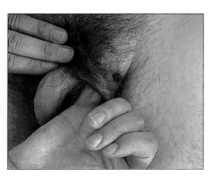

28.5 Diagnosis of a small inguinal hernia. The little finger of the examiner's hand is gently inserted at the level of the superficial inguinal ring by invaginating the scrotal skin, keeping the digit superficial in the inguinal canal and detecting a cough impulse on to the digit. Alternatively, inguinal and femoral hernias can be made more obvious by examining the patient in the standing position.

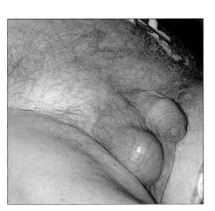

28.6 Indirect inguinal hernia in a male. The obvious swelling in the groin is differentiated from a femoral hernia as the hernia passes through the abdominal wall above and medial to the pubic tubercle. Swelling, cough impulse, discomfort and irreducibility are all features of an inguinal hernia.

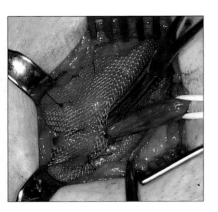

28.7 Lichtenstein repair. This is a **tension-free** repair which is associated with a 1% recurrence rate and uses a non-absorbable mesh sutured into the posterior wall. Splitting the mesh around the cord (fishtail fashion) tightens the deep ring with straining. Other methods of repair, such as Bassini and darn plication, may be associated with recurrence rates of up to 10%, whereas the Shouldice repair has a recurrence rate of 0.5–1%.

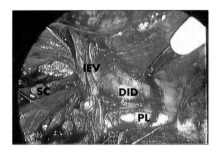 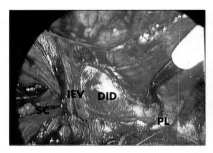

28.8 Laparoscopic pre-peritoneal approach to inguinal hernia. This shows the relationship in the pre-peritoneal space of the direct inguinal defect (DID) (*left*) and with extrinsic pressure applied (*right*) to the inferior epigastric vessels (IEV), the spermatic cord (SC) and pectineal line (PL). A prolene mesh, similar to that used for the Lichtenstein repair at open operation, is used to strengthen the posterior wall of the inguinal canal. This form of repair is useful for recurrent and bilateral hernia.

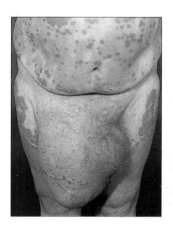 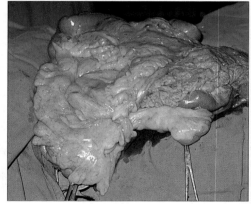

28.9 Direct inguino–scrotal hernia in a male. This 41-year-old man had a 5-year history of a progressively enlarging swelling in the groin (*left*). His main difficulty was that of micturating because of invagination of his penis in the scrotal skin. Other problems included the cosmetic appearance, obtaining trousers which would fit, and a complicating factor of extensive psoriasis. The hernial sac contained 90% of the small bowel, caecum, appendix, ascending colon and transverse colon (*right*). To effect reduction, an omentectomy, appendicectomy and orchidectomy were carried out. The excess sac was excised and closed. A Lichtenstein repair was carried out.

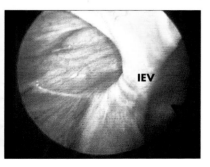

28.10 Incidental left indirect inguinal hernia at laparoscopy. Asymptomatic hernias are not infrequently found at laparoscopy carried out for other reasons, as shown here. The medial ridge of the defect is formed by the inferior epigastric vessels (IEV).

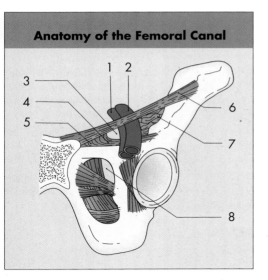

Anatomy of the Femoral Canal

1 Femoral vein.
2 Femoral artery.
3 Femoral ring.
4 Lacunar ligament.
5 Pectineal line.
6 Inguinal ligament.
7 Femoral nerve.
8 Obturator foramen.

28.11 Diagrammatic representation of the femoral canal. The femoral canal is an empty space containing lymphatic and adipose tissue. **Femoral herniation** occurs through the femoral ring which is bounded anteriorly by the inguinal ligament, medially by Cooper's ligament, posteriorly by the pectineal line and laterally by the femoral vein. **Strangulation** is more likely in a femoral hernia because of the fibro–osseus rigidity of the femoral ring.

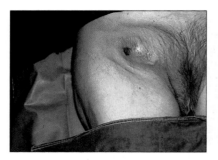
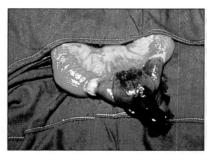

28.12 Femoral hernia. This is differentiated from an inguinal hernia as it passes through the abdominal wall below and lateral to the pubic tubercle. A cough impulse may be visible or palpable as a thrill. In this patient a fixed, tender and irreducible swelling (*left*) containing ischaemic ileum and a gangrenous Meckel's diverticulum (*right*) was present. The white rings around the bowel wall are ischaemic in nature; resection was necessary.

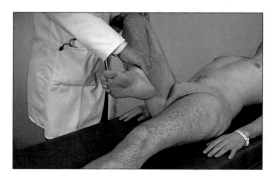

28.13 Diagnosis of an obturator hernia. This is a rare hernia and the diagnosis is made by a combination of clinical examination (exacerbation of the pain by hip flexion and internal [*top*] and external [*bottom*] rotation) with the radiograph appearances of a small bowel obstruction. Urgent laparotomy is indicated.

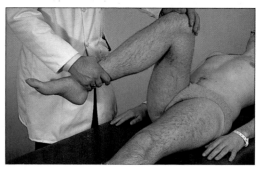

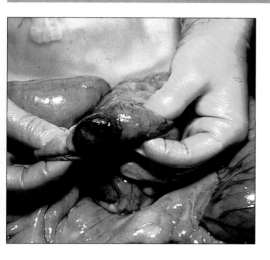

28.14 Richter's hernia in the obturator foramen.
This 47-year-old woman presented with a small bowel obstruction in a virgin abdomen associated with pain on hip flexion and rotation. A Richter's hernia occurs where only part of the circumference of the bowel wall has herniated through the hiatus (in this patient the obturator foramen) causing localised ischaemia.

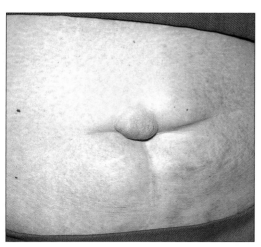

28.15 Para-umbilical hernia.
This predominantly affects obese multiparous women and is caused by a gradual weakening of the tissues around the umbilicus. The hernia passes through the attenuated linea alba and may be sited above or below the umbilicus. The sac is often multilocular and contains adherent omentum with loops of large or small bowel. This patient has had the hernia repaired previously and on this occasion by use of a polypropylene mesh.

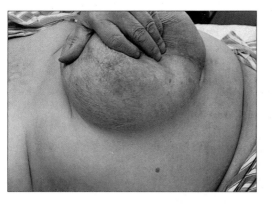

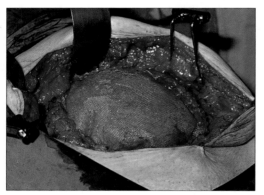

28.16 Incisional hernia.

This can occur in any surgical wound and is a diffuse protrusion of the peritoneum and abdominal contents through a weakened area in the wound. In this patient the hernia has occurred at the site of a previous midline laparotomy from 30 years earlier (**top**). **Precipitating factors** are principally, poor suture technique, wound dehiscence, chest and wound infection and post-operative distension. If it is broad based, this may not require surgical intervention but, should it become symptomatic, where the defect is small and the hernia large, surgery may be indicated. A prolene mesh has been used in this patient (**bottom**).

29.

SURGICAL GYNAECOLOGY

Principal Differential Diagnosis

Gynaecological causes of an acute abdomen are usually part of the differential diagnosis for acute appendicitis, and include:

- Ruptured ectopic pregnancy.
- Rupture of ovarian cyst.
- Torsion of ovarian cyst.
- Acute salpingitis.
- Pelvic inflammatory disease.

Bleeding from a ruptured Graafian follicle or corpus luteal cyst may cause abdominal pain. This usually occurs in the 15–25-year-old age group. There is sudden onset of pain in one or other iliac fossa. There may be associated nausea and vomiting. There are no systemic signs and pain usually settles within a few hours. Tenderness and guarding in the right iliac fossa can mimic acute appendicitis and a few patients bleed sufficiently to suggest rupture of an ectopic pregnancy. The pain may occur mid-menstrual cycle on a regular basis (**Mittelschmerz**). If there is doubt about the diagnosis, urine microscopy and urinalysis, laparoscopy and a pregnancy test can be carried out.

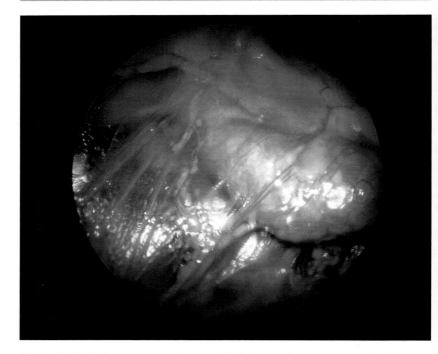

29.1 Pelvic inflammatory disease (PID). Acute salpingitis is most often due to *gonococcal* infection, but *Streptococci* and *Mycobacterium tuberculosis* may also be responsible. Urethritis, cervicitis and vaginal discharge occur 3–6 days following infection. The patient complained of lower abdominal pain associated with increased frequency of micturition, irregular menses, vaginal discharge, pyrexia and elevation of white cell count. On vaginal examination, the cervix was exquisitely tender and a high vaginal swab confirmed the diagnosis. Laparoscopy, which confirmed PID, was undertaken to exclude other pelvic pathology. Many pelvic adhesions were identified and the presence of a unilateral hydrosalpinx was indicative of the chronicity of the disease. (Reproduced with kind permission from Symonds EM, Macpherson MBA, *Color Atlas of Obstetrics and Gynecology*, Mosby–Wolfe, London, 1994.)

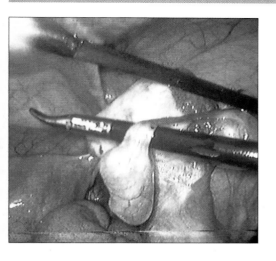

29.2   Fimbrial cyst torsion. Benign ovarian and fimbrial (as shown) cysts are common in women under 50 years of age, and may undergo torsion. This patient complained of sharp lower abdominal pain. A smooth, round and mobile fimbrial cyst on a long pedicle arising from the right ovary, found at laparoscopy, had undergone a 720° torsion. This was simply dealt with by excision.

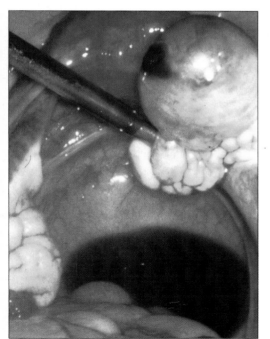

29.3   Bleeding ovarian cyst. These are relatively common and often present with a combination of sudden-onset lower abdominal and shoulder tip pain. The principal **differential diagnosis** includes PID and appendicitis. Laparoscopy demonstrated a bleeding right ovarian cyst with free blood in the pelvis.

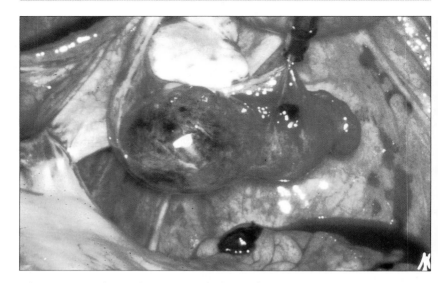

29.4 Ruptured ectopic pregnancy. The incidence is 1 in 200 pregnancies. The fallopian tube is the most common site, and rupture usually occurs after about 6 weeks of pregnancy. The symptoms are lower abdominal colic associated with vaginal bleeding. As the trophoblastic tissue penetrates the wall of the tube, there is sudden severe pain, blood loss and circulatory collapse. Abdominal pain becomes generalised and is associated with shoulder tip pain caused by diaphragmatic irritation from intra-peritoneal blood. Signs of pregnancy such as enlargement of the breasts and a history of a missed menstrual period may be present. The diagnosis is confirmed by laparoscopy or laparotomy, depending on the urgency, with removal of the ectopic pregnancy and fallopian tube preservation if possible. Following an ectopic pregnancy, there is a 10% risk of further ectopic pregnancy.

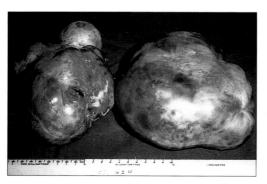

29.5 Kruckenberg tumours of the ovaries. Transcoelomic spread of gastric carcinoma has a predilection for the ovaries. Histological examination of these ovaries confirmed a typical signet ring appearance consistent with spread, 18 months following her gastrectomy.

Section 6

Vascular

30.

OCCLUSIVE ARTERIAL DISEASE

Epidemiology

Occlusive arterial disease is the single **most common cause of disability and death** in the Western world, often gives rise to life threatening complications, and frequently demands urgent surgical intervention. Symptomatic disease most commonly affects the leg, but may affect any vessel in the body. When arterial occlusion develops slowly, allowing collaterals to develop, the symptoms and signs are often insidious. By contrast, sudden arterial occlusion usually leads to catastrophic ischaemia and loss of limb and life in the absence of swift surgical revascularisation. By far the most important **risk factors** for the development of arterial occlusive disease are **smoking** and **diabetes**.

Pathology

Arterial occlusive disease is due to the development of **atherosclerosis** in which there is subintimal deposition of complex lipids and cellular elements (**atheroma**). As the atheroma develops, it impinges upon the lumen of the vessel forming a **plaque** which may form a haemodynamically significant stenosis. This pathological process may lead to **thrombosis, embolism** or **dissection**.

THROMBOSIS

Poor blood flow, together with plaque ulceration, lead to the exposure of blood to prothrombotic subendothelial tissues. This may lead to *in situ* thrombosis (platelets and red blood cells) and occlusion of the vessel.

EMBOLISM

Fragments of atheroma or thrombus (**embolus**) may be thrown off downstream and cause obstruction in the distal circulation (**embolisation**). Other common sources of embolus include the atria (in atrial fibrillation), the ventricles (mural thrombus from recent myocardial infarction), heart valves (prosthetic heart valves, cusp vegetations of infective endocarditis or rheumatic fever), and the aorta (abdominal aortic aneurysm).

DISSECTION

Ulceration of the arterial wall allows blood to drive a haemodynamic wedge through the media. A flap may be raised which obstructs flow and exposes blood to subendothelial tissues, so promoting thrombosis. Alternatively, the dissection may rupture outside the vessel or track back into the lumen creating a false lumen.

PERIPHERAL OCCLUSIVE ARTERIAL DISEASE

CHRONIC LIMB ISCHAEMIA

Intermittent claudication is the principal symptom of chronic limb ischaemia. It may be defined as ischaemic muscle pain coming on after walking and disappearing on rest, only to reappear when walking is resumed. In the UK, intermittent claudication affects approximately 5 per cent of men aged 60 years. It is a benign condition due to the body's ability to develop abundant collaterals, and less than 10 per cent of patients with claudication will ever require surgical intervention or amputation in the absence of continued smoking. Treatment consists of advice to **stop smoking**, to **lose weight**, and to **exercise** within the patient's pain limit. Co-existent medical conditions such as hyperlipidaemia, diabetes, hypertension and cardiac failure should be corrected where possible. Claudicants have a significantly reduced life expectancy from coronary and cerebral vascular events.

CRITICAL LIMB ISCHAEMIA (CLI)

This may be defined as ischaemic rest pain, requiring opiate analgesia and lasting at least two weeks, in association with an ankle pressure of less than 50 mmHg (or absent ankle pulses in the presence of diabetes). The two **cardinal features** of CLI are **rest pain** and **tissue loss** (ulceration/ gangrene). Once CLI develops, it is likely that the limb will be lost without active surgical intervention.

ACUTE LIMB ISCHAEMIA

Sudden arterial occlusion is usually caused by *in situ* thrombosis of a pre-existent atheromatous plaque or by embolus. There is sudden onset of rest pain followed by motor and sensory loss. On examination the '5 Ps' are sought: **pain, pallor, paraesthesia, paralysis** and `**perishing' cold**.

LOWER LIMB OCCLUSIVE ARTERIAL DISEASE

Clinical Assessment

Clinical assessment comprises history, examination and investigations (starting with the simplest and safest and progressing, if necessary, to the complex and invasive).

Differential Diagnosis

Nearly all arterial occlusive disease in the UK is directly attributable either to smoking or to diabetes. Other, relatively rare, diagnoses which should be borne in mind include:

- Arteritis:
    - Polyarteritis nodosa.
    - Takayasu's disease.
    - Scleroderma.
    - Systemic lupus erythematosis.
    - Giant cell arteritis.
- Fibromuscular hyperplasia.
- Trauma:
    - Thermal.
    - Blunt/penetrating.
    - Iatrogenic.
    - Intra-arterial injection of drugs.
- Buerger's disease.

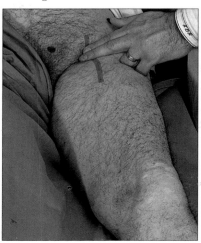

30.1   Palpation of the femoral artery. This pulse is easily felt below the mid-inguinal point. Pulses should be compared on either side. Reduced pressure on one side or a bruit on auscultation is indicative of aorto–iliac stenosis. An absent pulse denotes iliac occlusion. Bilateral absent pulses suggest aortic occlusion. The presence of a prominent or forceful pulse should alert the examiner to the presence of an aneurysm.

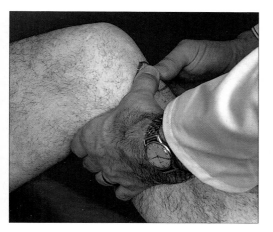

30.2 Palpation of the popliteal artery. With the knee flexed and the hamstring muscles relaxed, the thumbs of both examining hands are placed on the tibia tuberosity and the fingers of both hands palpate the popliteal fossa. Rotation of both hands together allows its detection just lateral to the mid-line. The popliteal artery trifurcates at its lower extent into three branches: posterior tibial, perineal, and anterior tibial arteries.

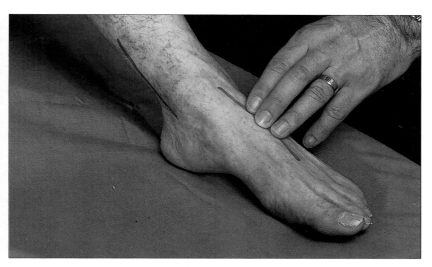

30.3 Palpation of the dorsalis pedis artery. This is a continuation of the anterior tibial artery which is felt on the dorsum of the foot just lateral to the tendon of the extensor hallucis longus. In about 10% of patients the dorsalis pedis is replaced as the major arterial inflow to the dorsum of the foot by the perforating perineal artery. This is not usually palpable but can be detected by hand-held Doppler ultrasound on the anterior aspect of the ankle mid-way between the tibia and fibula. The posterior tibial artery is in the groove posterior to the medial malleolus.

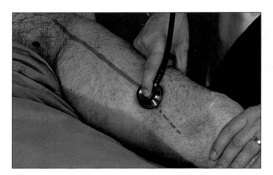

30.4 Auscultation of Hunter's canal. Superficial femoral artery stenosis in the adductor canal where the artery passes through the hiatus in the adductor magnus is often the earliest site of narrowing in lower limb peripheral arterial disease. On examination, a bruit may be heard at or below the adductor canal.

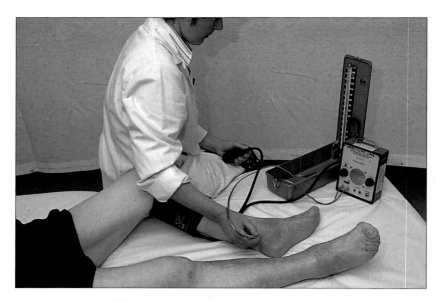

30.5 Doppler ankle pressures. The Doppler ultrasound probe is applied to the ankle vessels. Once a signal is obtained the blood pressure cuff is inflated around the calf. The pressure at which the signal in the artery disappears gives the perfusion pressure at the point at which the cuff is applied. It is customary to take the highest ankle pressure and to express this as a ratio with respect to the highest brachial pressure – the ankle:brachial pressure index (ABPI). In health the ABPI is at least 1.0. Patients with claudication normally have an ABPI of 0.6–0.9; with rest pain, 0.3–0.6; and with tissue loss < 0.3. Some patients, particularly diabetics, have heavily calcified arteries that cannot be compressed by the cuff; falsely elevated ankle pressures may then be obtained.

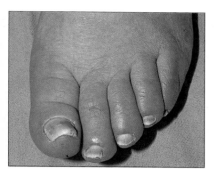

30.6 Chronic limb ischaemia.
Elevation of the leg results in marked pedal pallor due to inadequate perfusion against the forces of gravity, while, on dependency, as shown, the ischaemic foot becomes bright red, the so-called 'sunset foot', due to reactive hyperaemia. Patients with rest pain often note that pain is relieved by dangling the foot out of bed or by standing. The combination of **pallor on elevation** and **dependent rubor** is sometimes known as **Buerger's sign**.

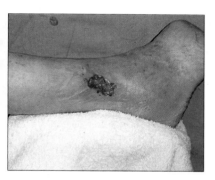

30.7 Ischaemic foot ulcer.
Ischaemic foot ulcers are usually found over pressure points such as the metatarsal heads, the malleoli, or the heel. Often there are clear features of arterial insufficiency such as in this patient who has previously undergone a transmetatarsal amputation for ischaemia. Few, if any, pure ischaemic ulcers will heal unless arterial inflow to the foot is improved by means of surgical revascularisation. The alternative is amputation.

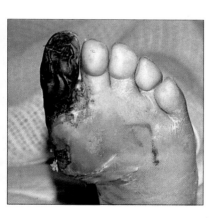

30.8 Gangrene.
Gangrene is the end-stage of peripheral vascular disease and inevitably requires some form of limited tissue debridement or formal amputation in combination with arterial reconstruction if the remaining wound is to heal. This patient has developed a necrotic hallux which required first ray amputation.

AORTO–ILIAC OCCLUSIVE ARTERIAL DISEASE

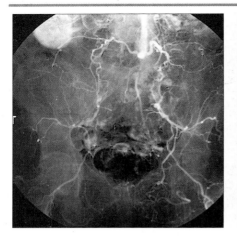 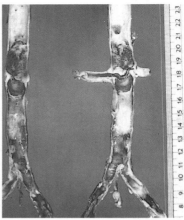

30.9 Aortic occlusion. Aortic occlusion may occur suddenly due to massive embolisation or to acute thrombosis of an abdominal aortic aneurysm. In these circumstances there is sudden and severe bilateral lower limb ischaemia and immediate surgical revascularisation by means of embolectomy or aortic bypass graft is necessary to save life. More commonly, as in this patient, a severely stenosed aorta develops thrombosis *in situ*. The presence of the well developed collaterals, seen in this angiogram (*left*), means that lower limb ischaemia is less severe. This patient succumbed from extension of the thrombosis, as shown in the pathological specimen (***right***).

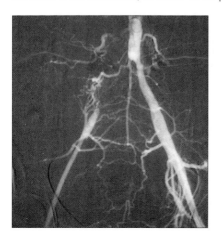

30.10 Iliac stenosis and occlusion before angioplasty. This patient presented with bilateral short distance thigh claudication and reduced femoral pulses. Angiography confirms the presence of a haemodynamically significant common iliac stenosis on the left and common iliac occlusion on the right suitable for percutaneous transcatheter balloon angioplasty (PTA) and stent placement.

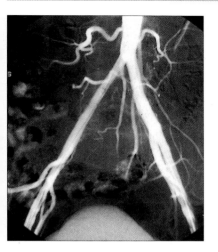

30.11 Iliac 'kissing' stent placement. Guide wires are placed up both iliac arteries following common femoral artery puncture under local anaesthesia, using the **Seldinger technique**. High pressure balloon catheters are then inflated in the diseased arteries, thereby enlarging or reconstituting the lumen on each side. Complications of this technique include dissection and thrombosis. To keep the arteries patent, expandable metal stents are now placed in each common iliac artery. Although the long-term patency of angioplasty with or without stenting is less than that of aortic bifurcation grafts, the former is associated with a serious morbidity and mortality of 1%; the latter up to 5%.

FEMORO–POPLITEAL OCCLUSIVE ARTERIAL DISEASE

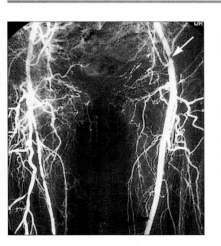

30.12 Common femoral artery (CFA) stenosis. This angiogram shows a CFA stenosis proximal to a patent femoro–popliteal bypass graft. The stenosis may be due to progression of proximal disease or to arterial clamp damage. This lesion is suitable for endarterectomy whereby the narrowing plaque is removed surgically. The artery is then closed, either directly or more commonly by means of a patch angioplasty.

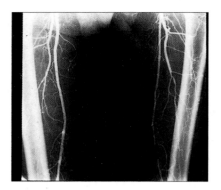

30.13 Superficial femoral artery (SFA) occlusion. This patient with a claudication distance of 200 m has a short left SFA occlusion at the adductor hiatus which is suitable for PTA. The profunda femoris system is well developed and relatively disease free. In general, the immediate and long-term results of PTA are better in the larger vessels and in stenoses rather than occlusions. Claudication most commonly affects the calf because arterial disease most often affects the femoro–popliteal segment.

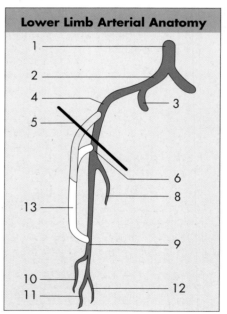

Lower Limb Arterial Anatomy

1 Aorta
2 Common iliac artery
3 Internal ilac artery
4 External iliac artery
5 Inguinal ligament
6 Common femoral artery
7 Superficial femoral artery
8 Profunda femoris artery
9 Popliteal artery
10 Anterior tibial artery
11 Peroneal artery
12 Posterior tibial artery
13 Graft

30.14 Femoro–popliteal bypass graft. This diagram shows the bypass of a block in the SFA by means of a femoro–popliteal bypass graft (white). If there is disease in the CFA as well, inflow for the graft can be taken from the iliac system (yellow). Bypass grafts can be fashioned with autogenous vein or with prosthetic materials – most commonly PTFE. The long-term patency of the former is generally better, especially when bypass grafts extend below the knee to the smaller crural vessels. If no usable vein is present, synthetic grafts may be used, but these, too, are more prone to infection.

INFRA-POPLITEAL OCCLUSIVE ARTERIAL DISEASE

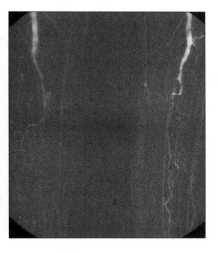

30.15   Crural disease. Crural (calf) arterial disease usually occurs as part of multi-segment disease. This angiogram shows the popliteal and crural vessels of both limbs to be severely stenosed or occluded. The patient presented with bilateral rest pain. No pedal vessels were detected by angiography or Doppler ultra-sonography. The patient underwent bilateral below-knee amputation, as the pedal vessels were occluded at surgery. In diabetics the pattern of disease is typically different in that crural disease may be associated with a relatively disease-free femoro–popliteal segment and pedal arch. In this case, bypass from the iliac or femoral segments to the pedal vessels may be successful.

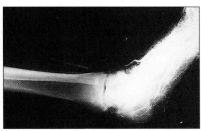

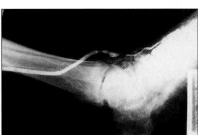

30.16   Distal bypass (on-table angiogram). In this diabetic patient the dorsalis pedis artery was seen to be patent on angiography (***top***). The vessel was explored and cannulated in the operating theatre and an on-table angiogram performed. This showed good flow of contrast into the foot. A vein bypass graft was therefore taken from the CFA to the dorsalis pedis artery. The completion angiogram (***bottom***) shows good flow of contrast down the vein graft, through the distal anastomosis and into the foot. Thus amputation was avoided.

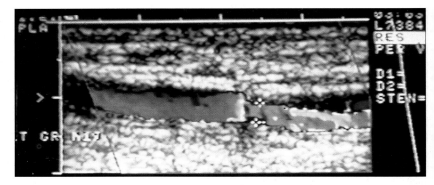

30.17   Vein graft stenosis (Doppler ultrasound). It is generally accepted that
bypass grafts fail due to the development of stenoses at the proximal and distal
anastomosis and, in the case of vein grafts, in the body of the graft itself. The value of
performing so-called graft surveillance is well accepted and the best way of demonstrating
graft stenosis is by Doppler ultrasonography. As the graft narrows the velocity of the blood
increases and this is detected as a colour change (red to yellow to green to blue).

ACUTE LIMB ISCHAEMIA

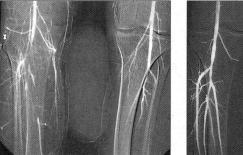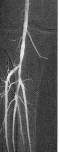

30.18   Popliteal embolus. Acute limb ischaemia is caused by embolus in about
one quarter of cases. Emboli usually lodge at branch points such as the CFA bifurcation
or the popliteal trifurcation, as shown in this angiogram (**left**). The standard treatment of
peripheral arterial embolus is embolectomy, during which the artery proximal to the
obstruction is opened and a balloon catheter passed through the embolus, the balloon
inflated, the catheter withdrawn, and the embolus extracted. Check angiogram on the
operating table confirms successful popliteal embolectomy in this patient (**right**). An
alternative treatment is to dissolve the clot by means of thrombolysis using streptokinase
or tissue plasminogen activator.

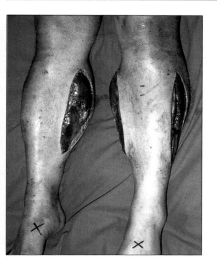

30.19 Fasciotomy. Revascularisation of damaged muscle following prolonged ischaemia leads to marked swelling. Unless the muscle is released from the constraints of the fascial compartments within the calf, this swelling may impede perfusion and lead to further muscle infarction. In order to prevent this complication, fasciotomy is commonly performed. This patient developed sudden acute bilateral lower limb ischaemia due to saddle embolus (an embolus lodging at the aortic bifurcation). Despite the gaping appearance of the wounds, fasciotomies are usually closed easily at about 10 days by means of direct suture or split skin graft.

UPPER LIMB ISCHAEMIA

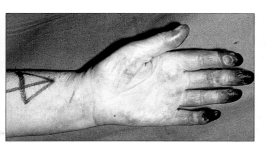
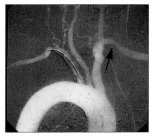

30.20 Distal embolisation. Upper limb ischaemia is relatively uncommon. The most common cause is embolus. This woman presented with gradual onset of fingertip necrosis on one hand due to the micro-embolisation of athermomatous material from a lesion in the subclavian artery (**left**). The arch aortogram shows left subclavian stenosis (**right**). There is slight stenosis of the right subclavian artery. The patient required amputation of the tips of the digits of her left hand and vein bypass of the subclavian lesion.

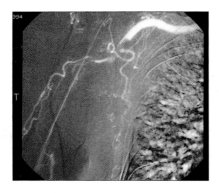

30.21 Axillary embolus. This patient in atrial fibrillation presented with sudden onset of pain, paraesthesia and paralysis in the right arm. Clinical examination revealed an absent brachial pulse, and urgent angiogram confirmed axillary embolus. There is a sharp cut-off in the lower axillary artery, and thrombus lying in the lumen. The patient was successfuly treated by means of brachial embolectomy and then warfarinised.

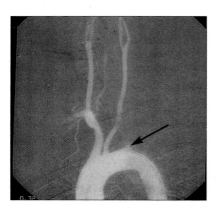

30.22 Subclavian steal syndrome. This arch aortogram shows complete occlusion of the left subclavian artery (*top*). The subclavian occlusion lies proximal to the origin of the left vertebral artery (*bottom*). Flow is via the carotid artery and the vertebral artery (VA) to the distal subclavian artery (DSA). Blood is thus stolen from the vertebral circulation leading to vertebro–basilar insufficiency: dizziness and syncope, classically occurring during muscular activity of the arm. The patient may also complain of weakness, tiredness and claudication of the upper limb.

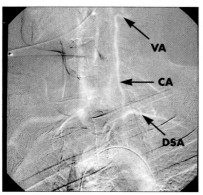

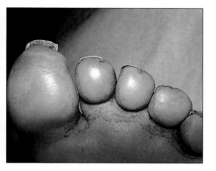

30.23 Frostbite. This is the most common thermal injury and is usually found in climbers, but not infrequently in homeless alcoholics and vagrants in whom the effects of cold lead to frostbite during the winter months. Treatment consists of reflex heating, analgesics, antibiotics and dextran infusion. Surgery is delayed until the area of dead tissue has become clearly demarcated, when debridement or, as in this patient, a transmetatarsal amputation, can be carried out.

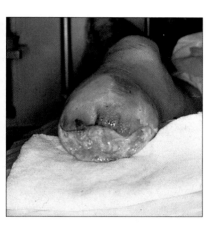

30.24 Below-knee amputation. This patient underwent below-knee amputation after failure to re-establish the peripheral circulation following femoro–popliteal graft occlusion. Aggressive reconstructive intervention is undertaken because amputation is associated with a 20% in-patient mortality, only 20% of patients will walk again and the total care costs presently amount to approximately £50,000 per patient. A high standard of nursing care, prudent surgical intervention and antibiotic usage is required in order to prevent secondary wound revision. Risk of stump breakdown can be reduced if thermal scanning of skin blood flow is carried out.

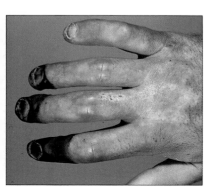

30.25 Ischaemic hand in a drug abuser. Peripheral vascular disease affecting the upper limb is much less common than that affecting the lower limb. Failed intravenous cannulation by drug abusers with injection of barbiturates into the artery may result in arterial spasm, or a trushing effect from particulate matter injected into the artery; and in this patient there is obvious gangrene of the fingertips. Treatment is expectant with systemic heparinisation. Where the digits or limb do not recover, amputation may be necessary.

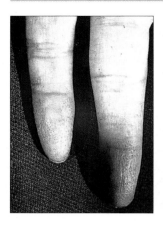
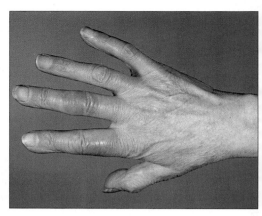

30.26 Raynaud's disease. Arterial vasoconstriction may be **primary** or **secondary** but, if severe enough, may cause fingertip necrosis (*left*). In its mildest form, the hands are particularly sensitive to thermal changes causing white, numb and painful fingers (*right*). Primary Raynaud's affects 5–10% of young women in temperate climates. No investigation is necessary and treatment consists of reassurance and avoidance of cold exposure. Secondary Raynaud's tends to occur in older people as a manifestation of scleroderma or systemic lupus, and can be associated with vibrating tools, beta-blocking drugs and blood dyscrasias.

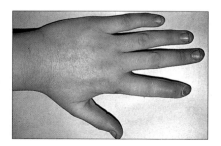

30.27 Thromboangiitis obliterans (Buerger's disease). This affects small arteries of the hands or feet producing occlusions, and is frequently accompanied by migratory phlebitis. It usually occurs in young males who are heavy smokers living in Mediterranean countries. The condition often remits if the patient stops smoking. Sympathectomy is helpful.

31.

ANEURYSMAL ARTERIAL DISEASE

Pathology

An aneurysm is an abnormal dilatation of an artery. **True aneurysms** are lined by endothelium and have media and adventitia in their walls. **False aneurysms** arise when the wall of the artery is pierced, resulting in haematoma which then liquefies leaving a cavity, lined by fibrous tissue, in continuity with the lumen. Anatomically, aneurysms may be **saccular** or **fusiform**. The principal complications of aneurysm are thrombosis leading to occlusion or distal embolisation, dissection and rupture.

THORACIC AORTIC ANEURYSM

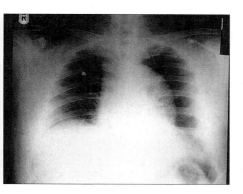
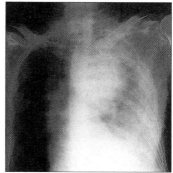

31.1 Thoracic aortic aneurysm. This **asymptomatic** lesion was detected incidentally on a chest radiograph (**left**). The patient was elderly with numerous medical problems, and no active treatment was proposed. Alternatively, the first presentation may be severe chest pain and signs of hypovolaemic shock indicative of thoracic **rupture**: the chest radiograph shows mediastinal widening, left chest opacification and marked tracheal deviation (**right**). Current evidence suggests that thoracic aortic aneurysms are at least as likely to rupture as abdominal aortic aneurysms (AAAs), and that, despite the high operative mortality and morbidity, operative repair should be considered in patients who are otherwise fit.

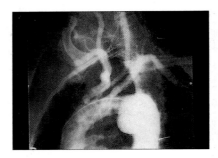

31.2 Thoracic aortography. In a patient being considered for operative repair of thoracic aortic aneurysm, CT scan and angiography should be performed to assess the extent of the aneurysmal dilatation and the state of the visceral, renal, and peripheral arteries. This angiogram shows a saccular aneurysm of the arch of the aorta at the origin of the left subclavian artery.

ABDOMINAL AORTIC ANEURYSM (AAA)

Although aneurysmal disease may affect virtually any artery in the body the most common type of aneurysm coming to the attention of vascular surgeons is the abdominal aortic aneurysm. Of these, 95 per cent affect the infra-renal aorta and 25 per cent extend into the iliac system. Approximately 10 per cent of patients with AAA also have a popliteal aneurysm, and in 40 per cent of such patients the aneurysm is bilateral.

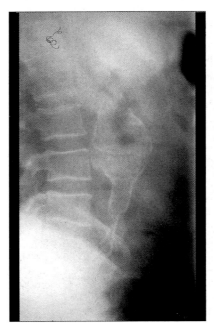

31.3 Abdominal aortic aneurysm (lateral abdominal radiograph). Approximately 60% of AAAs have enough calcium in their walls that they are readily seen on plain abdominal radiography. A lateral radiograph may be helpful if the diagnosis is suspected, particularly if the aneurysm is not evident on the antero–posterior view. The posterior wall of the AAA is applied to the spine and an estimation of its size as well as iliac and suprarenal extent can be made. Plain radiography does not provide any information with regard to the presence of rupture. The majority of aneurysms in the UK are due to age-related degeneration of the arterial wall. There also appears to be a strong, but as yet poorly understood, genetic component to the disease.

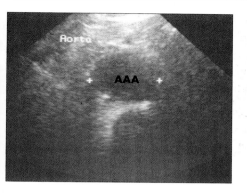 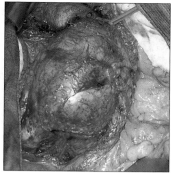

31.4 Abdominal aortic aneurysm (ultrasound scan). This is a useful diagnostic modality to measure AAA size and, as it is easily repeatable, it can also be used to monitor any increase in diameter (**left**). At operation, the aneurysm is isolated (**right**) and repair is undertaken by a straight tube or aorto–femoral graft. Screening programmes suggest that 5% of men in the UK aged 65 years have an AAA measuring greater than 4 cm in diameter (normal diameter 2.5–3.0 cm). Screening programs utilising ultrasonography have been advocated in the male population between the ages of 60 and 75 years at five-year intervals. Rapid increase in size of the aneurysm, pain, or a size greater than 6 cm, are indications for surgery.

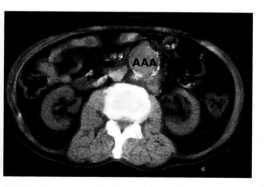

31.5 Ruptured abdominal aortic aneurysm (CT scan). This patient presented with a classic history of renal colic but, on examination, had a pulsatile mass. A ruptured AAA was suspected and confirmed on CT scanning. Although CT scan may be useful in this situation, there is a well recognised false positive and negative rate and the patient should be treated primarily on clinical grounds. Ruptured AAA is estimated to cause 1% of all deaths in males aged 65 years and over. Without surgery the condition is universally fatal; surgical repair is associated with a 30–70% operative mortality.

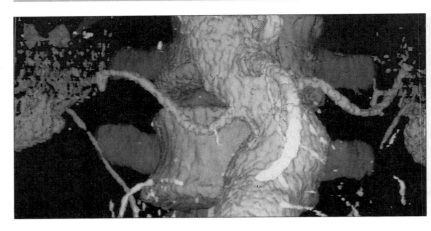

31.6 Abdominal aortic aneurysm (three-dimensional reconstruction from spiral CT). Modern computer software coupled to a spiral CT scanner allows three-dimensional reconstruction of the AAA to be produced. This precise information with regard to the morphology of the AAA is particularly useful when the patient is being considered for the relatively new technique of percutaneous stent grafting. Elective repair of AAA is associated with an operative mortality of less than 5%. It is important, therefore, that as many AAAs as possible are repaired prior to the occurrence of complications, notably rupture.

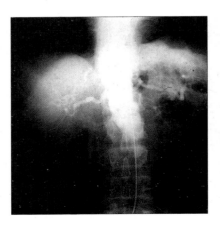

31.7 Suprarenal abdominal aortic aneurysm (aortogram). Approximately 10% of AAAs extend above the renal arteries as shown in this aortogram. Operative repair of such AAAs requires re-implantation of the visceral and renal arteries and is associated with an increased operative mortality when compared to infra-renal AAAs.

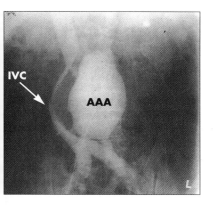

31.8 Aorto–caval fistula. This has arisen by spontaneous fistulation of an AAA into the inferior vena cava (IVC), and is demonstrated by angiography. On abdominal examination there was a pulsatile mass and a palpable thrill.

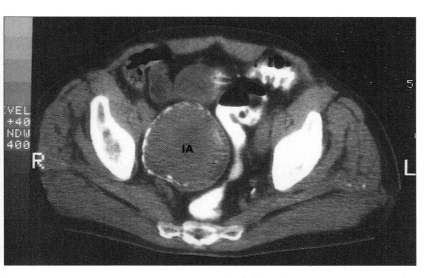

31.9 Iliac aneurysm. After AAAs, iliac aneurysms are the next most common site for aneurysmal dilatation. This patient presented with right groin discomfort. No abnormality was detected on abdominal examination but on digital rectal examination a pulsatile mass was felt on the right side. CT scanning confirmed the presence of a large aorto–iliac aneurysm (IA) compressing the rectum. For reasons unknown, aneurysms of the external iliac arteries are virtually unknown. Because of the high risk of rupture this patient underwent aorto–bi-iliac bypass grafting and made an uneventful recovery.

251

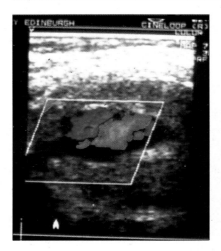
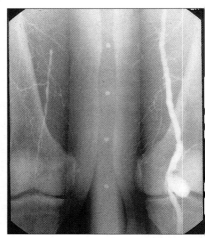

31.10 Popliteal aneurysm. This patient presented with a pulsatile mass in the abdomen and was found to have an AAA. On routine examination the left popliteal pulse was found to be widened. Doppler ultrasound scanning (*left*) confirms the presence of a large left popliteal aneurysm containing a narrow column of blood (blue/red) flowing through a large amount of thrombus (black areas). Angiography (*right*) demonstrates a saccular cavity containing flowing blood within the thrombus, filling the large fusiform aneurysm. Notice also the dilated and ectatic SFA artery above, which is typically found in these patients.

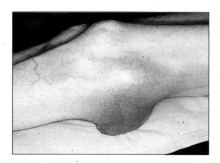
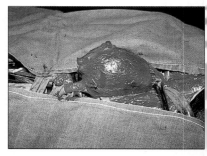

31.11 Popliteal aneurysm. Occasionally these aneurysms can reach considerable size and only present, as in this patient, when they interfere with function (*left*). At operation with the patient prone, the aneurysmal sac is isolated prior to excision and restitution of arterial continuity (*right*).

32.

VEINS AND LYMPHATICS

VARICOSE VEINS

In the UK, approximately 20 per cent of the adult population have varicose veins. The great majority of these arise from **valvular incompetence** within the superficial venous system (long and short saphenous veins) and the perforating veins that connect it to the deep venous system. Most patients with varicose veins are asymptomatic and never seek medical attention. Indications for intervention include **pain, phlebitis, ulceration, haemorrhage** and **cosmesis**.

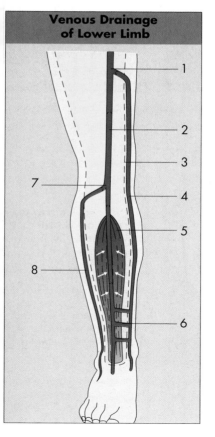

Venous Drainage of Lower Limb

32.1 Diagrammatic representation of the superficial and deep venous drainage of the leg. The long and short saphenous veins lie on the surface of the deep fascia. The long saphenous vein ascends anterior to the medial malleolus, posterior to the medial aspect of the knee, and then pierces the deep fascia 4 cm below and lateral to the pubic tubercle to join the common femoral vein. The short saphenous vein lies posterior to the lateral malleolus and passes posteriorly to the median line of the calf where it ascends to enter the popliteal vein. The superficial and deep venous systems are connected by a series of perforators, the largest of which are on the medial side of the thigh and lower calf.

1 Sapheno–femoral junction
2 Deep vein (femoral)
3 Deep fascia
4 Superficial vein (long saphenous)
5 Calf pump
6 Perforating veins
7 Sapheno–popliteal junction
8 Short saphenous vein

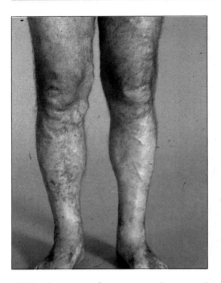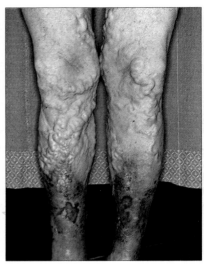

32.2 Long saphenous varicose veins. The middle-aged patient pictured (***left***) has marked varicose veins affecting the right long saphenous system. He presented with a general discomfort and feeling of fullness in both legs, symptoms which were worse on standing. The other patient (***right***) presented with gross bilateral varicose veins and associated ulceration.

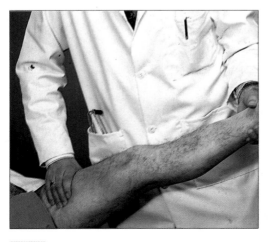

32.3 Trendelenburg test of sapheno–femoral incompetence. The leg is elevated and a rubber tourniquet applied just at or below the sapheno–femoral junction. The patient is then asked to stand. The veins fill slowly from arterial inflow but quickly from venous reflux. If venous distension below the tourniquet is controlled, as in this patient, the site of reflux must be above it. By removing the tourniquet at different levels, the pattern of incompetence can be mapped.

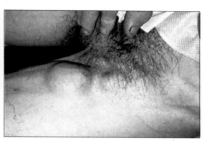 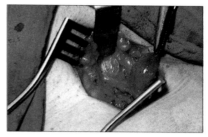

32.4 Saphena varix. This is a 'blow out' at the sapheno–femoral junction (**left**) and should be considered in the **differential diagnosis** of groin swellings. Care must be taken at operation to dissect out the varix as it is often thin-walled (**right**). Standard treatment of long saphenous incompetence is ligation of the sapheno–femoral junction, above-knee stripping and multiple stab avulsions/ligations.

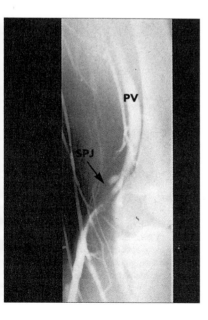

32.5 Short saphenous varicose veins. Approximately 20% of patients with varicose veins have predominantly short saphenous varicosities. This venogram shows the sapheno–popliteal junction (SPJ) and provides the surgeon with a 'road-map' of where to commence the dissection in the popliteal fossa. This is important as the level of the junction can be very variable and is difficult to localise by means of clinical examination alone. **Doppler ultrasound** can also be used for this purpose and in those patients who are obese or have recurrent varicosities. Failure to identify and ligate the true junction is the most common cause of recurrent varicosities. Minor varicosities below the knee may be initially dealt with by **injection sclerotherapy** with ethanolamine or sodium tetradecyl-sulphate. Compression is maintained for three weeks. (PV = popliteal vein.)

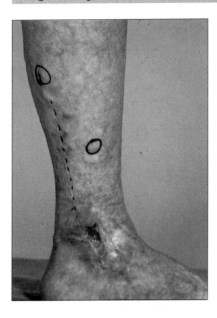

32.6 Calf perforators. It is generally taught that, in health, perforating veins only transmit blood from the superficial to the deep venous systems and that reflux is prevented by the presence of valves. Furthermore, it is believed by some that, in the presence of deep venous hypertension, high pressures can be transmitted to the skin leading directly to venous ulceration. The pathophysiology is almost certainly far more complex than this and the importance of ligating perforating veins in the management of venous ulceration is the subject of much debate.

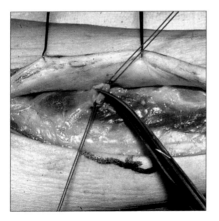

32.7 Perforator ligation.
Perforating veins can be divided percutaneously, either through stab incisions or following formal dissection of the subfascial plane. The disadvantage of the former is that it can be difficult to localise perforators clinically; and of the latter that it entails a major wound through skin that is often diseased and heals poorly. A more recent innovation is endoscopic subfascial ligation of perforators, where a small endoscope is passed into the subfascial plane under tourniquet control. This largely avoids the problems associated with the percutaneous approach.

CHRONIC VENOUS INSUFFICIENCY AND ULCERATION

Approximately 1 per cent of the adult population in the UK have chronic skin changes and ulceration of the calf, due to **venous hypertension**. Opinions vary as to whether pure superficial venous incompetence can lead to varicose ulceration; most authorities believe that a degree of deep venous or perforator incompetence is required in most patients. Deep venous incompetence is the result of previous **deep venous thrombosis** (DVT) or, as in varicose veins, due to **primary valvular insufficiency**. The aetiology of the latter condition is poorly understood. A small proportion (10 per cent) of patients also have a degree of venous obstruction due to previous DVT, and these patients often have severe skin disease. Valvular incompetence and obstruction lead to sustained venous hypertension in the lower limb. Although several theories have been proposed, it is as yet unclear how this leads to the skin changes of lipodermatosclerosis and ulceration.

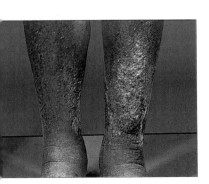

32.8 Lipodermatosclerosis (varicose eczema). Increased capillary permeability is thought to lead to the deposition of fluid, plasma proteins, red blood cells and haemosiderin within the skin.

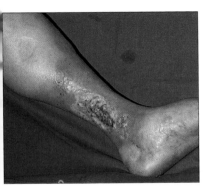

32.9 Chronic venous ulceration. The ulcer is typically situated in the gaiter area, on the medial aspect of the leg, is shallow, and is surrounded by varicose eczema. The cost to the National Health Service (in the UK) of caring for these patients each year is presently estimated at between three and six hundred million pounds. Treatment comprises care of the ulcer, the use of compression stockings, and surgical intervention to the associated varicosities if this is indicated and once the ulcer has healed.

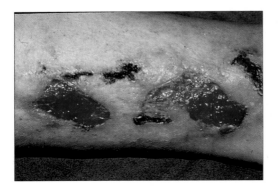

32.10 Arterial disease. The second most
common cause of leg ulceration is ischaemia, which
often coexists with venous disease in the elderly
population. The detection of arterial impairment is
vital as the conventional treatment for venous
ulceration is compression therapy. In the presence of
ischaemia this can precipitate further tissue damage
over pressure points, as shown here.

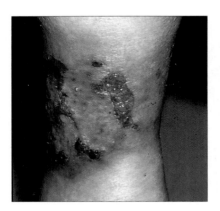
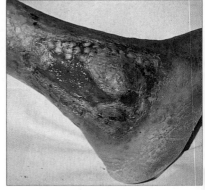

32.11 Skin grafting to varicose ulceration. Approximately 60% of venous
ulcers can be healed by 6 months of multilayer compression bandaging that aims to
apply graduated compression to the leg, pressure being highest (30–40 mmHg) at the
ankle and lowest at the knee (10–20 mmHg). Once the ulcer base is healthy and
granulating, healing can be hastened by means of split skin grafting (**left**), or pinch skin
grafting (**right**) as shown here.

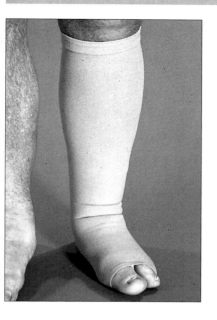

32.12 Compression bandaging.

Once the ulcer is healed, recurrence is prevented by the application of graduated compression support stockings. In the presence of arterial disease compression therapy is limited, and patients must be treated by means of bed rest and leg elevation, together with arterial reconstruction where possible. Unusually ulcers are so intractable that primary amputation is required.

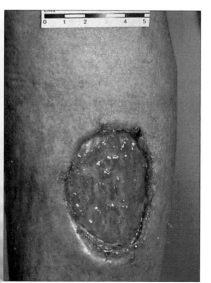

32.13 Malignant ulcer.

Approximately 1% of all leg ulcers are malignant, most commonly being squamous cell carcinomas. The clinician should be suspicious if the ulcer is at an unusual site, is punched out with a rolled margin, and is not associated with evidence of arterial or venous disease such as lipodermatosclerosis. Long-standing venous ulceration predisposes to malignant change (**Marjolin's ulcer**). Failure to heal should also prompt biopsy to exclude malignancy. Treament is by excision followed by skin grafting.

DEEP VENOUS THROMBOSIS (DVT)

Without thrombo-embolic prophylaxis, deep venous thrombosis (DVT) may develop in the legs of up to 20 per cent of patients after major surgery. The great majority of DVTs are asymptomatic until a piece of thrombus breaks off and embolises to the lung as a pulmonary embolus (PE). PE is one the most common causes of sudden death after surgery. Venous thrombosis is favoured by slow flow, intimal damage and hypercoagulable blood.

Peri-operative risk factors associated with an increased risk of DVT and PE include:
• Previous DVT or PE.
• Advanced age.
• Malignant disease.
• Varicose veins.
• Obesity.
• Polycythaemia.
• Thrombocytosis.

Prevention of DVT depends upon identification of 'at risk' patients, and the institution of prophylactic measures, such as:
• Graduated compression stockings.
• Intermittent pneumatic compression of calves per-operatively.
• Electrical stimulation of calf muscles per-operatively.
• Early mobilisation.
• Low-dose heparin.

Heparin is given at a dose of 5000 IU twice daily by subcutaneous injection, commenced at least two hours per-operatively, and has been shown by randomised controlled trial to reduce the incidence of fatal postoperative PE.

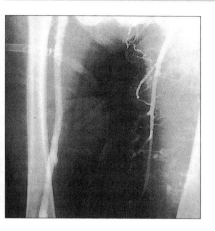
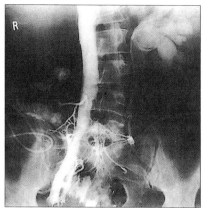

32.14 Bilateral ascending venography for deep venous thrombosis (DVT). This venogram shows occlusion of the left superficial femoral vein (*left*), and the iliac system with a tongue of thrombus lying within the inferior vena cava (*right*) which occurred after urinary tract surgery. Clinical examination is unreliable in the diagnosis of DVT and pulmonary embolus (PE) and must be supplemented by some form of radiological investigation. Doppler scanning may be able to detect thrombus in the femoro–popliteal segments, although it is unreliable in the calf and iliac veins. The risk of PE is greater the further up the leg the thrombus extends. It is vital, therefore, that the upper limit of the thrombus be visualised in every case.

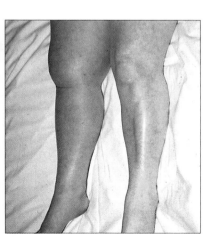

32.15 Iliofemoral DVT. The clinical photograph shows a swollen right leg due to iliofemoral venous thrombosis. The cause of this patient's thrombosis was external compression of the iliac vein from bladder carcinoma. If the diagnosis of PE is suspected, chest radiograph, ventilation perfusion (VP) scanning and pulmonary angiography should be undertaken. Evidence of PE is found in 40% of asymptomatic patients and is a marker for increased risk of further PE.

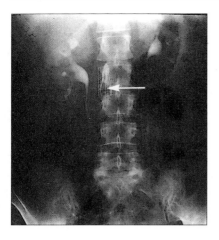

32.16 Inferior vena caval anti-embolic filter. Patients with proven pulmonary embolus (small and/or multiple), or 'free-floating tails' of thrombus in the iliac or caval veins, are at substantial risk of massive pulmonary embolus. Insertion of a caval filter via the femoral vein into the inferior vena cava (IVC), as shown here, prevents embolic material reaching the pulmonary circulation. Indications for placement of an IVC filter include further PE while fully heparinised and the presence of absolute contraindications to the use of heparin (e.g. recent stroke). The development of venous gangrene is now extremely rare.

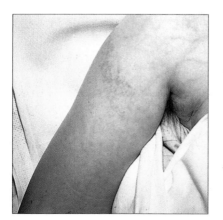

32.17 Spontaneous axillary vein thrombosis. This healthy young patient complained of the sudden onset of discomfort and heaviness in his arm, which is cyanosed and displays venous engorgement. Venous collaterals have developed over the shoulder and anterior chest wall. In other patients, there may be a previous history of intermittent venous obstruction in the limb due to a mechanical cause at the thoracic outlet. These include cervical rib, abnormal muscle or ligamentous bands at the inner border of the first rib, or a narrow interval between the clavicle and the first rib.

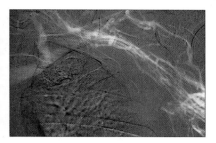

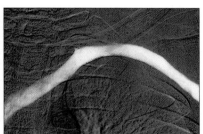

32.18 Axillary vein thrombosis (venography). The venogram (*top*) defines the occlusion with thrombus in the distal axillary vein and demonstrates the presence of multiple collaterals. The patient was successfully treated with thrombolytic therapy with early resolution of symptoms (*bottom*). Further venography showed the presence of a venous web which was treated by means of percutaneous balloon angioplasty and placement of a stent. The patient was anticoagulated for 6 months and the stent remained patent.

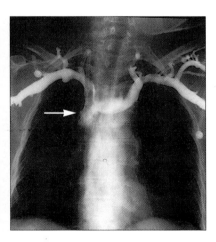

32.19 Central venous catheter-related thrombosis of the superior vena cava. Parenteral nutrition or pressure monitoring may cause thrombosis in the great veins of the neck. The superior vena caval thrombosis demonstrated here is associated with a right internal jugular Hickman line.

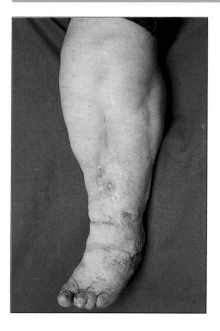

32.20   Primary lymphoedema.

This is a familial condition caused by reduction in the number of lymphatics and hypoplastic development of the lymphatic system. It usually affects females, may be unilateral or bilateral, may affect upper or lower limbs and is particularly noticeable after exercise or exposure to warmth, and in the pre-menstrual period. The swelling is initially soft and pitting but the high protein content of the retained fluid gradually leads to fibrosis and hyperkeratosis. The diagnosis is confirmed by lymphangiography. Treatment is directed at limb elevation, intermittent pneumatic compression, and graduated elastic compression stockings. These patients do not develop limb ulceration.

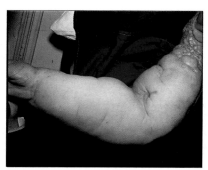

32.21   Secondary lymphoedema.

A secondary cause should be sought where lymphoedema develops late in life or where there is a clear history of an antecedent condition which involves lymphatic trunks and lymph nodes becoming obstructed by tumour, recurrent infection, infestation with filariasis, surgery or radiotherapy. This slide shows arm lymphoedema consequent upon axillary node involvement with carcinoma of the breast.

Section 7

Endocrinology

33.

THYROID AND PARATHYROID

THYROID

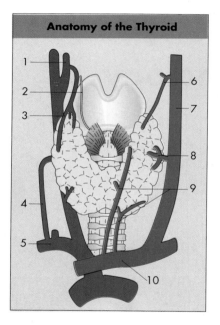

Anatomy of the Thyroid

1 External carotid artery
2 External laryngeal nerve
3 Superior thyroid artery
4 Inferior thyroid artery
5 Subclavian artery
6 Superior thyroid vein
7 Internal jugular vein
8 Middle thyroid vein
9 Inferior thyroid veins
10 Brachiocephalic vein

33.1 Anatomy. The thyroid gland is situated anteriorly and laterally in the lower part of the neck at the level of the 5th, 6th and 7th cervical vertebrae. There are right and left lobes connected by a narrow isthmus which lies over the 2nd and 3rd tracheal rings. The gland weighs approximately 30 g and derives its blood supply from the superior and inferior thyroid arteries. The inferior thyroid artery runs upwards and immediately behind the carotid sheath to the posterior aspect of the lower third of the gland. A short distance from the gland, the artery passes behind or in front of the recurrent laryngeal nerve or it may branch around it. The recurrent laryngeal nerves course upwards in the groove between the oesophagus and the trachea to enter the larynx. Lymphatic drainage of the gland is laterally to the deep cervical chain and anteriorly to the pre-tracheal mediastinal nodes.

Diagnosis
- General examination (including assessment of thyroid function).
- Examination of thyroid gland and cervical lymph nodes.
- Total and free serum thyroxine (T4) and tri-iodothyronine (T3).
- Thyroid stimulation hormone (TSH) levels.
- Thyroid auto-antibodies.
- Plain cervical radiology.
- Chest radiograph, with thoracic inlet view if necessary.
- Thyroid ultrasonography.
- ^{99m}Tc-labelled sodium pertechnetate or ^{125}Iodine uptake.
- Fine-needle aspiration cytology.

Classification of Thyroid disease.

Simple
- Diffuse hyperplastic goitre.
- Nodular goitre.
- Diffuse toxic goitre (Graves' disease).

Toxic
- Toxic nodular goitre.
- Toxic nodule.

Neoplastic
- Benign.
- Malignant.

Thyroiditis
- Granulomatous thyroiditis (De Quervain's disease).
- Auto-immune thyroiditis.
- Riedel's thyroiditis.

Other
- Acute bacterial thyroiditis.
- Chronic bacterial thyroiditis (tuberculosis and syphilis).
- Amyloid goitre.

Causes of Goitre
- Physiological: puberty; pregnancy; menopause.
- Endemic: lack of iodine in the diet.
- Goitrogenic agents.
- Thyrotoxicosis.
- Hashimoto's disease.
- Infective thyroiditis.

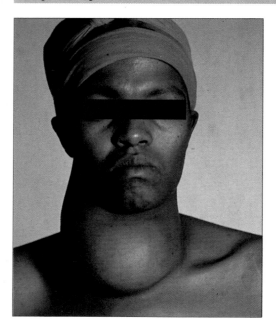

33.2 Simple goitre.
Goitre is a visible or palpable enlargement of the thyroid and, in this patient, was asymptomatic. The surface is smooth, with soft to firm consistency. Most goitres occur in euthyroid individuals (normal thyroid function) but can arise in hypothyroid or hyperthyroid individuals.

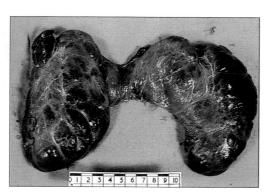

33.3 Nodular goitre. Pathological specimen of a thyroid which has become diffusely enlarged. The follicles become filled with colloid (colloid goitre) and, later, multiple nodular areas develop, as shown here, while other areas show degenerative changes with cyst formation, recent or old haemorrhage and calcification. Although most multi-nodular goitres are asymptomatic, haemorrhage into one of these nodules may cause pain and rapid enlargement.

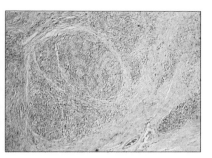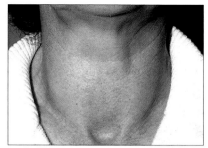

33.4 Hashimoto's thyroiditis. Hypothyroidism secondary to autoimmune thyroiditis is shown in this histological section (***left***). A diffusely enlarged gland shows marked lymphocytic infiltration around destroyed follicles. Although the patient can be euthyroid or thyrotoxic with a mild degree of goitre (***right***), symptomatic hypothyroidism is common in this condition which most commonly affects post-menopausal females (female to male ratio of 10:1).

HYPOTHYROIDISM

The **cardinal symptoms and signs** of hypothyroidism are tiredness, mental lethargy, cold intolerance, increase in weight, constipation, menstrual disturbance, carpal tunnel syndrome, slow pulse rate, dry hair and skin, cold extremities, peri-abdominal puffiness, hoarse voice, slow movements, slow reactions and ankle jerks.

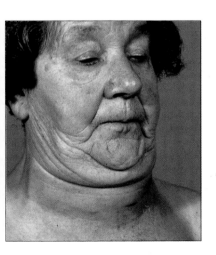

33.5 Myxoedema. This term should be reserved for very advanced forms of hypothyroidism in which the facial appearance is of supraclavicular puffiness, with a malar flush, expressionless facies and an acute yellow tinge to the skin.

HYPERTHYROIDISM

The **cardinal symptoms and signs** of hyperthyroidism are weight loss despite a good appetite, heat intolerance, diarrhoea, excitability and anxiety, moist, warm skin, excessive sweating, tachycardia, palpitations, thyroid tremor, lid lag and proptosis, pre-tibia myxoedema, myopathy, finger clubbing, menstrual irregularities and relative infertility. Atrial fibrillation may be present and, because of the increased vascularity, a bruit may be audible over the thyroid.

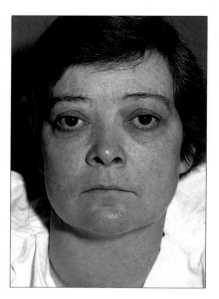

33.6 Primary thyrotoxicosis (Graves' disease). This is an auto-immune disease in which TSH receptors in the thyroid gland are stimulated by circulating immunoglobulins. Graves' disease accounts for 75–80% of cases of thyrotoxicosis occurring in young females (female to male ratio of 8:1) and there is a strong genetic predisposition. The **differential diagnosis** is that of thyrotoxicosis arising in a nodular goitre or a toxic adenoma.

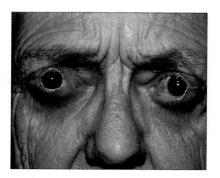

33.7 Eye signs associated with thyrotoxicosis. Progressive exophthalmos is a distressing and fortunately rare condition. Despite ablation of the thyroid, the condition may progress with proptosis, deterioration of vision, corneal ulceration, chemosis, papilloedema, ophthalmoplegia and panophthalmitis. Lateral tarsorrhaphy has been carried out in this patient.

THYROID NEOPLASMS

Classification

Benign
- Follicular adenoma.

Malignant
- Primary:
  - Papillary (60%).
  - Follicular (17%).
  - Anaplastic (13%).
  - Medullary carcinoma (6%).
  - Lymphoma (4%).
- Secondary:
  - Local infiltration.
  - Metastatic (carcinoma of breast and bronchus).

Fifty per cent of **cystic swellings** result from colloid degeneration or are of uncertain origin because of the absence of epithelial cells in the lining. Most of the remainder are attributable to degeneration of a follicular adenoma. 10–15 per cent of cystic swellings are histologically malignant on fine-needle aspiration. About 80 per cent of discrete swellings are cold on radio isotope scan. Only 20 per cent of these are malignant and use of this criterion as an indication for surgical intervention is inappropriate. Although hot nodules are very seldom malignant, this possibility cannot be ignored. Routine isotope scanning has been abandoned in favour of fine-needle aspiration, although the former is still necessary in the investigation of hyperthyroidism.

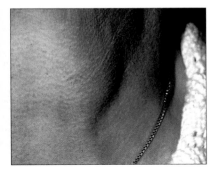

33.8 Follicular adenoma. This presents as a solitary nodule and can only be differentiated from follicular carcinoma by histological examination. There is no invasion of the capsule or peri-capsular blood vessels in the adenoma and treatment is therefore by lobectomy.

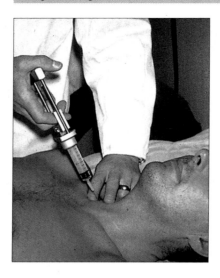

33.9 Fine-needle aspiration (FNA) of a follicular carcinoma. This male patient in his late twenties presented with a rapidly enlarging nodule in the right lobe of the thyroid. FNA demonstrated a follicular pattern. At operation, frozen section confirmed the presence of malignancy and he proceeded to lobectomy with excision of the isthmus. Lymph node metastases are rare but blood-borne spread to lungs, bone or liver occurs in 20% of patients. The 10-year survival rate is 50%.

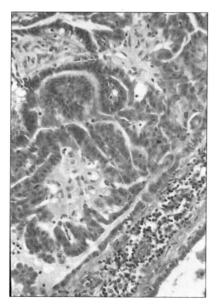

33.10 Papillary carcinoma. Histological sectioning of a thyroidectomy specimen from a patient in her mid-twenties confirms the FNA findings of a papillary carcinoma. This lesion occurs in the 15–40 age group, presents as a solitary lump, is relatively slow growing, but metastasises to deep cervical lymph nodes. As the disease is commonly multi-focal, a total thyroidectomy is carried out with removal of obviously involved lymph nodes, although radical neck dissection is no longer favoured. Thyroxine replacement is required and the 10-year survival rate is almost 90%.

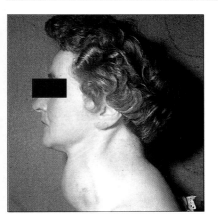

33.11 Anaplastic carcinoma. This patient presented with a rapidly growing neck swelling causing hoarseness, dyspnoea and dysphagia through local pressure effects. Fine-needle aspiration confirmed the presence of an anaplastic carcinoma and radiotherapy was given. The one-year survival rate is less than 30%.

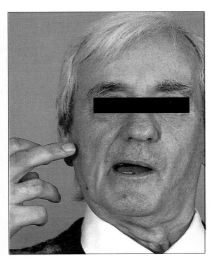

33.12 Chvostek's sign.
Hyperexcitability of motor neurone groups due to a fall in serum calcium concentration is the result of damage to the parathyroid glands during thyroidectomy. Treatment consists of intravenous calcium gluconate with subsequent administration of oral calcium and vitamin D (cholecalciferol) and, if necessary, correction of magnesium deficiency. Other **complications of thyroidectomy** include haemorrhage, superior laryngeal nerve damage resulting in temporary weakness of the voice, damage to the sympathetic chain during ligation of the inferior thyroid artery causing Horner's syndrome, hypothyroidism and keloid formation in the neck.

PARATHYROID

Of the two pairs of parathyroid glands, the **superior** ones are applied closely to the posterior aspect of the upper lobes of the thyroid at the level of the cricoid cartilage and are constant in position. The **inferior** glands are usually closely applied to the posterior surface of the lower lobes within their fascial sheath. Occasionally they may be found below the thyroid in the upper mediastinum or within the thymus gland. The parathyroids secrete parathormone which maintains the plasma and tissue levels of calcium. Recurrent urinary calculi may be the presenting feature of hyperparathyroidism as a result of the hypercalcaemia which will result in polyuria and eventual renal failure if left untreated (**35.13**). Isolated hypercalcaemia must be differentiated from parathyroid disease by excluding metastatic bone disease and other causes such as excessive absorption of calcium, excessive breakdown of bone and ectopic secretion of parathormone-like substances.

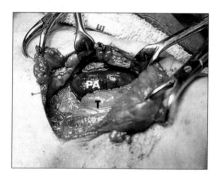

33.13   Primary hyper-parathyroidism. This operative photograph shows a solitary parathyroid adenoma (PA). These benign tumours may reach 10 times the size of a normal parathyroid. In 2% of cases, more than one gland is affected. Diagnosis is made on the basis of raised serum calcium and parathormone levels. **Differential diagnosis** includes secondary and tertiary hyperparathyroidism, and parathyroid carcinoma. (T=Thyroid)

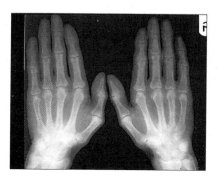

33.14   Osteitis fibrosa cystica of the fingers. Bone damage is now rarely seen, but gross demineralisation, subperiosteal bone resorption, cysts in long bones and the moth-eaten appearance of the skull are common manifestations of overactivity of the parathyroid gland. Other clinical manifestations include neurological and psychiatric symptoms and acute pancreatitis.

34.

ADRENAL

Each adrenal gland weighs approximately 4 g and rests on the superior, anterior and medial aspects of the superior pole of the corresponding kidney. It has a deep yellow colour and a firm consistency which enables the gland to be differentiated from the adjacent fat.

Its component parts include an **adrenal cortex** which is made up of three layers: the **zona glomerulosa**; the **zona fasciculata**; and the **zona reticularis**, which secretes **mineralocorticoids** (principally aldosterone), **glucocorticoids** (principally hydrocortisone) and **androgenic** and **oestrogenic hormones**. These steroid groups overlap in their actions and account for the variable clinical presentation of the patient with overactivity of the adrenal cortex.

The internal component (**adrenal medulla**) produces **catecholamines** in a ratio of 80 per cent adrenaline to 20 per cent noradrenaline, and is supplied by pre-ganglionic sympathetic nerves.

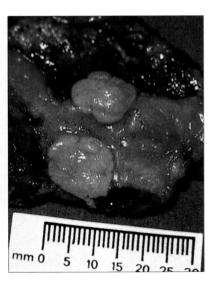

34.1 Primary aldosteronism (Conn's syndrome). This pathological specimen shows a cortical adenoma which is benign and occurs most commonly in young or middle-aged women. The patient presented with hypertension due to retention of sodium, muscular weakness due to hyperkalaemia and alkalosis. The diagnosis was confirmed by a low serum potassium, elevated aldosterone levels and low plasma renin levels which distinguish it from aldosteronism that is secondary to disease of the cardiovascular system, kidneys or liver.

HYPOADRENOCORTICISM

Adrenocortical insufficiency may present with muscular weakness and low blood pressure. There is irregular dusky pigmentation of the skin, due to deposits of melanin appearing at points of pressure, pigmentation of mucous membranes, particularly of the mouth. If the disease becomes fully established, acute adreno-cortical insufficiency may result. This condition arises from lymphocytic infiltration of the zona reticularis. The aetiology is autoimmune in 60 per cent (**Addison's disease**), with tuberculosis, metastatic carcinoma and amyloidosis accounting for the remaining 40 per cent.

In acute adrenal failure, haemorrhage into the skin progresses rapidly into the purpuric areas. This condition, **Waterhouse–Friderichsen syndrome**, is associated with shock and is characteristic of the patient presenting with massive bilateral adrenal cortical haemorrhage associated with meningococcal septi-caemia. Other causes include severe septicaemia in infants and young children and severe haemorrhage or burns in the adult. Treatment with antibiotic therapy, hydrocortisone, oxygen and intensive care monitoring is mandatory.

HYPERADRENOCORTICISM

Overactivity of the adrenal cortex may be due to **hyperplasia** of the gland, a functioning **cortical adenoma** or **carcinoma**, and may be secondary to a **basophil pituitary adenoma**.

Pituitary tumours are the most common cause of Cushing's syndrome (80 per cent) and a few cases may arise from **inappropriate** or **ectopic adrenocortico-trophic hormone** (ACTH) production (e.g. pancreatic or bronchial carcinoma).

Diagnosis
- General examination.
- Plasma cortisol, ACTH and aldosterone levels, urinary steroid excretion.
- Dexamethasone suppression test (distinguishes between adrenal and pituitary causes).
- Ultrasonography.
- CT or iodocholesterol scanning.
- Selective adrenal vein catheterisation.

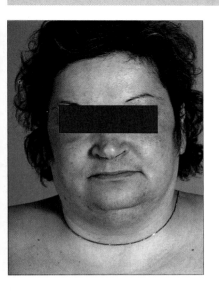

34.2 Cushing's syndrome. This middle-aged patient has the typical appearances of hypersecretion of hydrocortisone and corticosterone. There is central distribution of fat ('moon face', 'buffalo hump'), hirsutism, acne and striae. This condition is associated with amenorrhoea, hypertension, diabetes and osteoporosis.

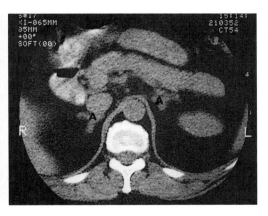

34.3 Cushing's syndrome. This CT scan shows hyperplasia of both adrenal glands (A) associated with an ACTH-secreting pituitary adenoma. There are high ACTH levels and urinary cortisol excretion is suppressed by dexamethasone. Bilateral adrenalectomy requires the patient to be maintained on lifelong mineralocorticoid and steroid replacement therapy. Alternatively, microsurgical removal of the pituitary adenoma or implantation of Yttrium-90 has been used, but these are associated with a high incidence of recurrence and can be reserved for those patients who develop Nelson's syndrome.

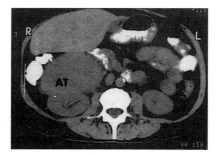

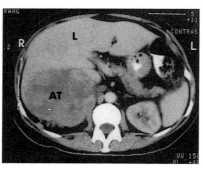

34.4 Cushing's syndrome. These CT scans demonstrate a large right adrenal tumour (AT) (***top***) infiltrating the liver (L) (***bottom***). A chest radiograph confirmed the presence of diffuse small pulmonary metastases and the patient's symptoms were poorly controlled with metyrapone and aminoglutethamide before her death.

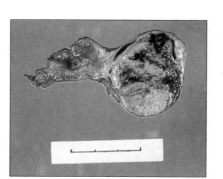

34.5 Cushing's syndrome. The cortical adenoma shown on this pathological specimen accounts for 20% of instances of Cushing's syndrome, and may be bilateral. Serum ACTH levels are low with elevated plasma cortisol levels and 24-hour urinary-free cortisol excretion. Localisation of adenomas is by CT or MRI scanning. Infrequently, a rare adrenal carcinoma can produce syndromes identical to either Conn's or Cushing's syndromes.

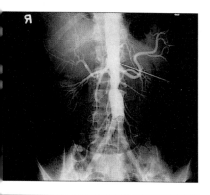

34.6 Non-functioning adrenocortical adenoma. This arteriogram (***top***) demonstrates a large, asymptomatic, space-occupying lesion above the displaced right kidney in a patient being investigated for peripheral vascular disease. This specimen (***bottom***) was removed and shows a well defined encapsulated tumour which, on histology, proved to be more cystic than solid.

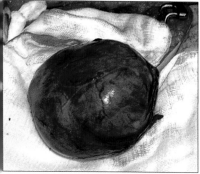

ADRENAL MEDULLARY TUMOURS

Neoplasms arising from sympathetic neurones are either **ganglion neuromas** or **neuroblastomas**. The former are generally benign while the latter are highly malignant tumours found in children.

Tumours arising in the adrenal medulla from the chromatin cells are **phaeochromocytomas**, 10 per cent of which are malignant, 10 per cent occur outside the adrenal and 10 per cent are part of the multiple endocrine neoplasia syndrome.

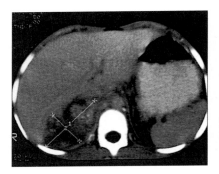 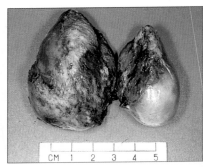

34.7 Neuroblastoma. Patients may present with an abdominal mass, weight loss, failure to thrive, abdominal pain and distention, fever or anaemia, as in this 5-year-old boy. If excess catacholamine production is present, hypertension, flushing, sweating and general irritability may be found. The diagnosis was confirmed by CT scanning (*left*). Iodobenzylguanidine is metabolised by neuroblastoma cells and may be used in scanning for the detection of metastatic or residual disease. The pathological specimen (*right*) is of the most common solid tumour in infancy and childhood arising from the neural crest.

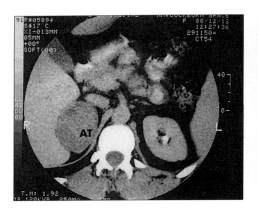 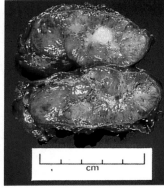

34.8 Phaeochromocytoma. The diagnosis is made by measurement of free catecholamines and the catecholamine metabolite, vanillylmandelic acid (VMA), in a 24-hour collection of urine. The tumour AT is readily localised by CT scan in this patient (*left*). Approximately 10% of lesions are bilateral, malignant (necessitating radical adrenalectomy, **right**), extra-adrenal, multiple, familial or occur in children. The secretion of catecholamines may cause headache, palpitations, sweating, blurred vision, weakness, pallor and paroxysmal hypertension. The **differential diagnosis** is hyperthyroidism, hypercalcaemia, acute anxiety state and carcinoid syndrome.

Section 8

Urology

35.

KIDNEY AND URETER

The **cardinal symptoms and signs** of urinary tract disease are **renal pain** radiating from the renal angle around the loin into the groin, to either the testis or the labia; **ureteric pain** with a similar distribution but intermittently exacerbated due to colic; and **lower abdominal pain**, possibly associated with **bladder obstruction**. Urinary frequency, poor stream and dribbling, urgency, incontinence, dysuria, haematuria, strangury, renal mass, lower abdominal mass and prostatic enlargement on digital rectal examination, are all indicative of urinary tract disease.

Principal Differential Diagnosis of a Renal Mass

Solid
- Renal cell carcinoma.
- Transitional cell carcinoma.
- Nephroblastoma.
- Metastatic tumours.
- True sarcoma.
- Benign tumours (lipoma, haemangioma, leiomyoma, hamartoma, lymphangioma).
- Retroperitoneal teratoma.
- Xanthogranulomatous pyelonephritis.
- Renal carbuncle.
- Angiomyolipoma.

Cystic
- Simple cyst.
- Multiple cysts.
- Polycystic disease.
- Cystadenoma.
- Perinephric abscess.
- Dermoid.
- PUJ obstruction.

Other Differential Diagnosis
- Adrenal tumour.
- Liver enlargement: benign/malignant tumours;cystic disease.
- Mucocele of gallbladder (right-side).
- Splenic enlargement (left-side).
- Colonic carcinoma.

Diagnosis

- General examination and urinalysis.
- Ultrasonography.
- Intravenous urography (IVU).
- CT scanning.
- Angiography.
- Chest radiograph (neoplastic disease).
- Retrograde pelvi–ureterography.
- Ureteroscopy.
- Urea, creatinine and electrolytes.
- Creatinine clearance.
- DMSA, DPTA and MAG 3 renal isotope scanning.
- Urine cytology.
- Urine culture and microscopy.

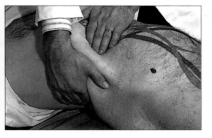

35.1 Bimanual palpation of the kidneys. The kidneys are not usually palpable in a normal patient unless the patient is very thin. Using the posterior hand, the kidney is brought forward to be felt by the anterior hand using the method known as 'ballotment'. Renal enlargement is not usually detected unless lesions are of substantial size.

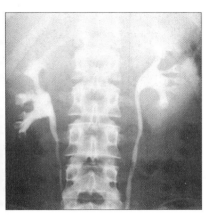

35.2 Intravenous urogram (IVU). This investigation shows excretion of contrast, which demonstrates the relationship of the kidney and ureters to the spinal column and is *not* a test of renal function. The hila of the right and left kidneys lie above and below the L_1/L_2 vertebral level. The ureters lie over the tips of the transverse processes, cross the pelvic brim at the sacro–iliac joint, and pass towards the ischial spines before turning back towards the mid-line to enter the bladder base in the trigone.

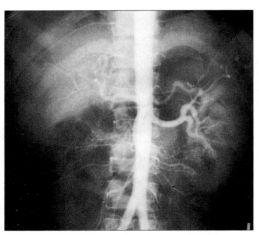

35.3 Solitary kidney.
This congenital abnormality, demonstrated by angiography, has an incidence of 1 in 2000. It is therefore important that, where a nephrectomy is considered necessary, it is established that the contra-lateral kidney is present and functioning.

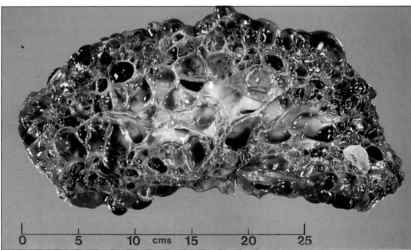

35.4 Polycystic disease. Polycystic kidneys may not become manifest until the third and fourth decades, when the patient may present with a symptomatic mass, progressive renal failure and/or hypertension. Bleeding into cysts may cause acute pain and is dealt with by simple needle aspiration. If enlargement is such that it splints the diaphragm or interferes with space for successful transplantation, unilateral nephrectomy is indicated. Alternatively, polycystic disease may be detected by antenatal ultrasonography, or the infant may present with enlarging masses in both flanks. Progressive renal failure usually results and renal transplantation offers the only prospect of normal renal function.

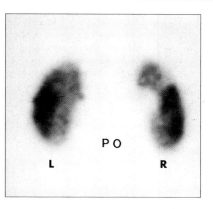

35.5 Simple renal cyst (DMSA scan).

Patients may complain of persistent renal angle pain and tenderness, recurrent urinary tract infection, sudden pain due to haemorrhage into a cyst, and, rarely, an abdominal swelling. Assessment of renal function by ^{99m}Tc-labelled dimethyl succinic acid (DMSA) scan demonstrates a filling defect in the parenchyma of the right kidney which was confirmed on ultrasound. Ultrasound-guided aspiration is the initial treatment but recurrent cysts are managed by open or laparoscopic excision or marsupialisation.

P O

L   R

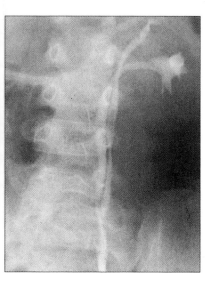

35.6 Ureteric duplication.

This is a common abnormality with complete duplication of upper and lower moieties which are associated, in some cases, with a ureterocele.

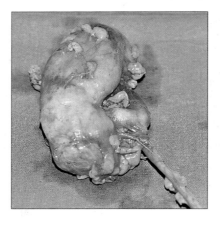

35.7 Pelvi–ureteric junction (PUJ) obstruction. This pathological specimen shows a grossly dilated renal pelvis with stenosis at the pelvi–ureteric junction which is crossed by aberrant lower pole vessels. These lesions are often detected by antenatal ultrasonography where the principal **differential diagnosis** is a simple cyst. Early operation by pyeloplasty is performed after birth to improve calyceal drainage, resulting in reduced parenchymal loss and improved renal function. Occasionally, PUJ obstruction presents in adults.

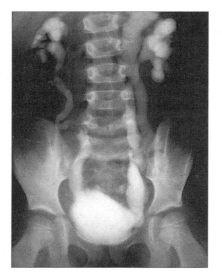

35.8 Vesico–ureteric reflux (micturating cystogram). This 8-year-old girl presented with recurrent urinary tract infections and occasional incontinence. There is marked vesico–ureteric reflux which, if untreated, will cause renal impairment. She underwent cystoscopic STING (submucosal teflon injection) procedure on two occasions to reduce reflux at the ureteric orifices. Re-implantation of ureter(s) may be necessary if the STING procedure is unsuccessful.

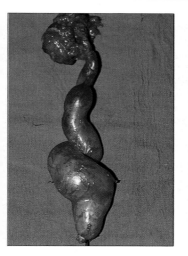

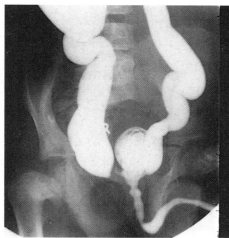

35.9   Renal dysplasia and hydroureter. There is gross dilatation of the ureter associated with a dysplastic, poorly functioning kidney (**left**). Depending on aetiology of hydronephrosis/hydroureter, this condition may be unilateral or bilateral (as shown on the IVU, **right**), congenital or acquired.

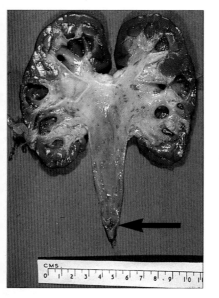

35.10   Chronic pyelonephritis. This 33-year-old, who had a history of recurrent urinary tract infection secondary to vesico–ureteric reflux, underwent nephrectomy because of recurrent sepsis and systemic hypertension. Recurrent stone formation was a feature of the presentation (arrow indicates stone in ureter). DMSA scanning indicated that the kidney only contributed 5% to the overall renal function.

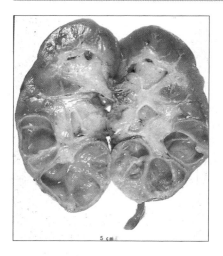

35.11 Renal tuberculosis. Early caseating lesions are found near the junction of the cortex and medulla (in this patient, at the lower pole). These enlarge, caseate and then rupture into a calyx, eventually producing extensive destruction of the renal parenchyma (as demonstrated). As the ureter becomes infiltrated and thickened, obstruction leads to pyelonephrosis. The diagnosis was confirmed by staining and culture of mycobacteria in early-morning specimens of urine. Although tuberculosis is relatively uncommon, its frequency is increasing again, particularly among immigrant populations.

Predisposing Factors to Stone Formation

- **Inadequate drainage:** renal obstruction and stagnation; bladder diverticulum; prolonged immobilisation or recumbency.
- **Excess of normal constituents:** hyperparathyroidism; prolonged immobilisation and widespread skeletal metastases (calcium); gout, leukaemia and polycythaemia (uric acid).
- **Presence of abnormal constituents:** urinary tract infection producing epithelial slough as a focus for stone formation; foreign body (catheter, suture material); hyperkeratosis of epithelium (vitamin A deficiency); cystinuria.

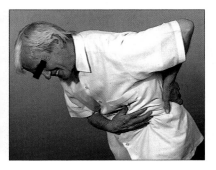

35.12 Renal colic. This patient is suffering from severe left ureteric colic, which was relieved by intravenous pethidine. Haematuria and proteinuria are frequently present on urinalysis. Plain abdominal radiography will show a radio-opaque calculus in 80% of patients. In the UK, 80% of the stones are mixed calcium oxalate/phosphate; 10% are magnesium ammonium phosphate stones with a variable proportion of calcium. The remainder are uric acid (95%), cystine (1–4%) and xanthine (1%) stones. In **elderly patients** presenting with a history of renal colic, the **first exclusion diagnosis** should be a **ruptured aorta aneurysm**.

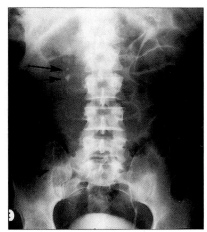

35.13 Ureteric calculus. This IVU shows impaction of the calculus at the level of the pelvic brim, which was responsible for this patient's presentation. There are two other stones in the right renal pelvis. The stone passed spontaneously, as occurs in the majority of patients. During their passage renal calculi can be arrested at three points: the pelvi–ureteric junction, the pelvic brim and at the ureteric orifice in the trigone.

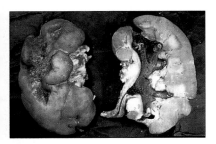

35.14 Staghorn calculus. Few patients now reach this stage of gross stone disease which requires nephrectomy or open stone extraction. The treatment of renal calculi has radically changed over the last decade with the widespread introduction of extracorporal shock wave lithotripsy, percutaneous nephrolithotomy and ureteroscopic stone destruction (by laser, electrohydraulic lithotripsy or ultrasonic probe), with or without dormia basket extraction.

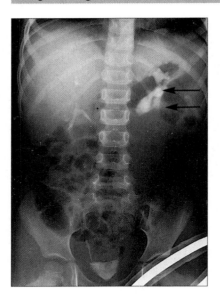

35.15 Blunt renal trauma (IVU). A fall from a swing caused this child's haematuria and left-sided pain. The IVU shows extravasation of contrast from the left renal pelvis. This injury was treated conservatively with complete resolution of symptoms.

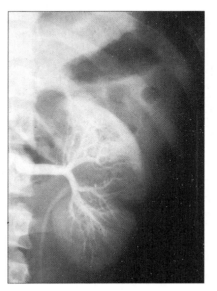

35.16 Renal trauma (angiography). This 27-year-old male who was involved in a road traffic accident had evidence of shock and haematuria on admission. Following resuscitation, renal angiography showed a parenchymal tear in the left kidney which was observed and did not require surgical intervention.

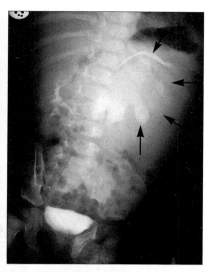

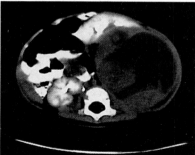

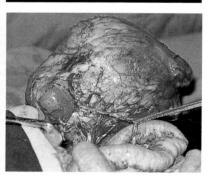

35.17 Nephroblastoma (Wilm's tumour). This 3-year-old child was admitted with a large abdominal mass and a low-grade pyrexia. Wilm's tumour is derived from embryonic mesodermal tissue and is bilateral in 5–10% of patients. Intravenous urography (*top*) is essential, as the principal **differential diagnosis** is an adrenal neuroblastoma. A CT scan confirms the diagnosis with a large space-occupying lesion in the left flank (*middle*). Transabdominal nephrectomy is shown here with wide excision of the mass carried out after preliminary ligation of the renal pedicle (*bottom*). The ureter has a rubber sling around it. The 5-year survival rate is now 80% with combination radio- and chemotherapy.

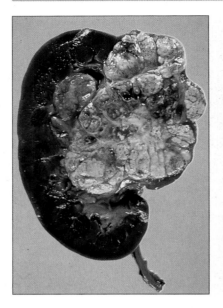 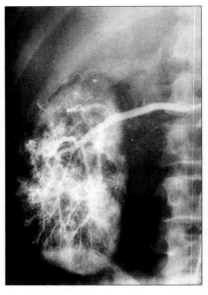

35.18   Renal cell carcinoma. This is the most common malignant tumour of the kidney (two to three times more common in men); its maximal incidence is in the 6th to 8th decades (*left*). There is early spread of the tumour into the renal pelvis causing haematuria and invasion of the renal vein, with possible tumour emboli. Angiography (*right*) showing the tumour circulation may also be used pre-operatively to embolise larger tumours. This is one of the five common tumours to spread to bone, the other four being lung, breast, thyroid and prostate.

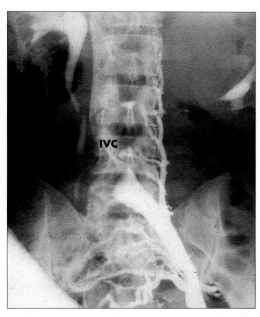

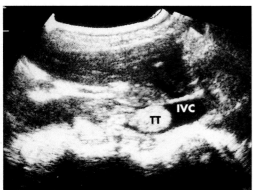

35.19 Renal cell carcinoma. Because of its propensity to spread along the renal vein into the inferior vena cava (IVC) from the left kidney as shown (***top***), leading to tumour thrombus (TT) extension superiorly and inferiorly along the IVC, it is necessary to prevent embolus by temporarily cross-clamping, opening the IVC and removing the tumour. Inferior cavography does not always reliably detect IVC tumour, and ultrasonography (***bottom***) may provide more accurate information. If the upper extent is supra-diaphragmatic then echocardiography is necessary. **Local presenting features** include: haematuria, 'clot colic', a renal mass and rarely a varicocele. **Systemic symptoms**, possibly due to secretion of erythropoietin, renin, parathormone and gonadotrophins, include: pyrexia, coagulopathy, polycythaemia, and abnormalities of plasma proteins and liver function.

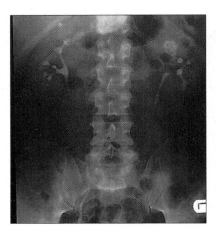

35.20 Transitional cell carcinoma of the renal pelvis. Urothelial tumours of this nature affecting the renal pelvis (2%) or ureter (1%) are much less common than their bladder counterparts (97%). A small left renal pelvis lesion is shown on this IVU in a patient being investigated for haematuria and pain. Treatment is by nephro–uretrectomy.

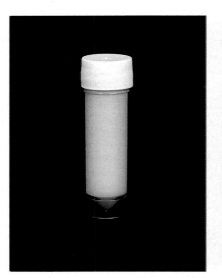

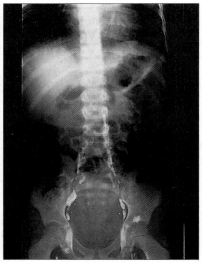

35.21 Chyluria. This milky urine (*left*) is taken from an 8-year-old boy who presented with a 3-year history of progressive colour change in his urine. Although a lymphangiogram (*right*) did not confirm the presence of a pyelo-lymphatic fistula, the patient underwent renal pedicle stripping of lymphatics with successful resolution of his symptoms.

36.

BLADDER AND PROSTATE

The **cardinal symptoms and signs** associated with disease of the lower urinary tract are: lower abdominal pain associated with a distended bladder; pain associated with cystitis; frequency of micturition, difficulty, hesitancy, poor stream and dribbling associated with bladder outlet obstruction; strangury due to the severe pain associated with the passage of a stone; haematuria; nocturia; faecaluria and pneumaturia; urgency; incontinence; a palpable bladder; and enlarged tender or irregular prostate gland on rectal examination.

Diagnosis
- General examination and urinalysis.
- Ultrasonography.
- Cystography.
- CT scanning.
- Cystoscopy.
- Urodynamic studies.
- Urine cytology.
- Urine culture and microscopy.

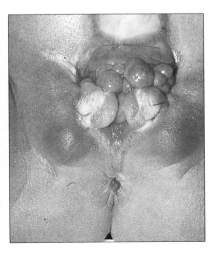

36.1   Ectopia vesicae. This is an uncommon congenital malformation. The bladder mucosa is exposed to the anterior abdominal wall with urine constantly excreted from the exposed ureteric openings. Symphysis pubis separation is present, resulting in a waddling gate due to pelvic instability. Ureteric reflux of urine is common. Reconstruction of the bladder is extremely difficult and, if not possible, an alternative procedure is urinary diversion. The patient's quality of life is poor, owing to the high incidence of secondary renal infection.

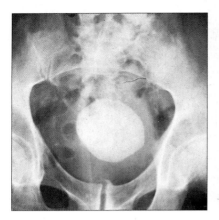
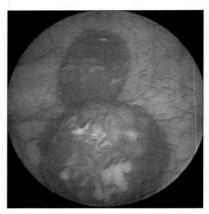

36.2 Bladder calculi. A large bladder calculus is seen as an incidental finding on plain abdominal radiography (***left***). More commonly, calculi seen at cystoscopy (***right***) are usually the result of recurrent urinary tract infections. Although these are easily dealt with by mechanical lithotripsy and bladder washout, the underlying cause of urinary tract outflow obstruction should be sought.

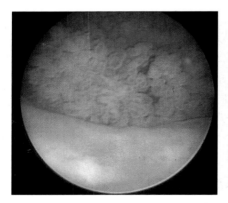
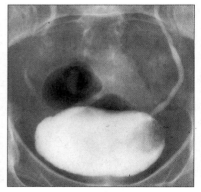

36.3 Transitional cell carcinoma of the bladder. This large papillomatous growth was resected transurethrally in a patient presenting with painless haematuria (***left***). He was initially investigated by an IVU which demonstrated an irregular filling defect in the bladder (***right***). Consider a **differential diagnosis** of adenocarcinoma, squamous cell carcinoma, rhabdomyosarcoma or an invasive colonic adenocarcinoma.

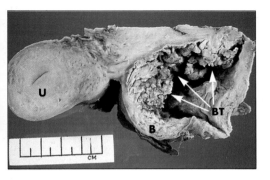

36.4 Bladder carcinoma (cystectomy specimen). This female patient underwent cystoscopic surveillance and resection of recurrent bladder tumours for several years. The tumour was not controllable by this method. CT scanning of the pelvis suggested invasion of the bladder wall. The extensive bladder tumour (BT) shows invasion of the surrounding structures. U = uterus; B = bladder.

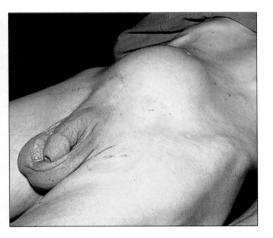

36.5 Chronic retention of urine. Examination of this elderly patient demonstrated a lower abdominal mass which was smooth, dull to percussion and arising out of the pelvis to the level of his umbilicus. Similar findings in a woman would suggest the **differential diagnosis** of an ovarian cyst or uterine fibroids. The most common cause of urinary retention, which can be acute or chronic, is benign prostatic hypertrophy.

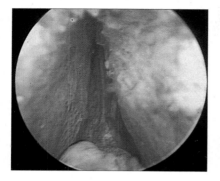

36.6 Benign prostatic hypertrophy.
Urethroscopic assessment of prostatic lateral lobar enlargement is shown where the mons verumontanum is the key landmark, seen at the 6 o'clock position. Pre-operatively, urinary flow rate studies, ultrasonographic assessment of post-voiding residual urine volumes and serum biochemistry for evidence of renal impairment are performed. Serum prostate specific antigen (PSA) is assayed to exclude malignancy but, following transurethral resection of the prostate (TURP), histological examination of the prostatic chips is mandatory.

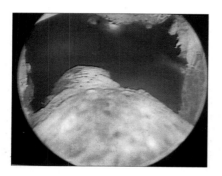

36.7 Prostatic bed after TURP.
Approximately 30 g of prostate were resected in order to improve urinary flow, and the wide open bladder neck is clearly seen. Transurethral resection of the prostate has largely replaced open prostatectomy, which is reserved for massive prostatic hypertrophy. Medical treatments and thermal or laser ablation of the prostate are presently being evaluated.

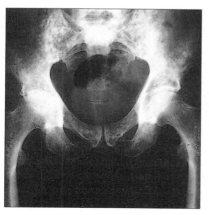

36.8 Prostatic carcinoma metastases.
Radiography of the pelvis shows characteristic osteosclerotic secondaries, confirmed by radio-isotope bone scan, from prostatic cancer which is the second most common malignancy in males. It is uncommon before 60 years of age. The diagnosis may be made by rectal examination (the gland is hard and irregular), incidentally at histology of prostatic chips, and from a presentation due to malignant dissemination with weight loss, back pain, anaemia and an elevated PSA. The diagnosis was confirmed by a grossly elevated PSA and positive histology.

37.

URETHRA AND PENIS

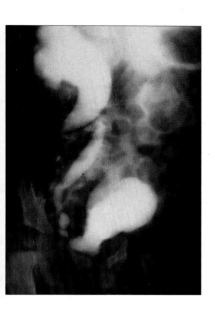

37.1 Urethral valves. Urethral valves (demonstrated at urethroscopy) occur in boys and are found in the posterior urethra. Delay in the diagnosis is not uncommon. When urine is tentatively passed, they balloon up like a parachute so that great pressure is required to overcome the obstruction. The presentation may be dribbling of urine, and renal impairment from the obstructive uropathy causing failure to thrive. The contrast study shows the gross dilatation of the urinary tract. The principal **differential diagnosis** is a urethral diaphragm, or stricture, and bladder neck obstruction. Treatment is by valvotomy.

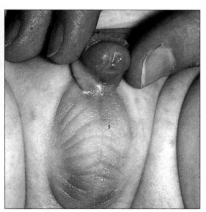

37.2 Glandular hypospadias. This is a common malformation in which the urethral opening is on the ventral surface of the glans. Where meatal hypospadias is present, this condition may be missed because of the small blind pit. The prepuce is always abnormal and, instead of encircling the glans, it is gathered as a hood on the dorsal surface. Some degree of cordee is present causing the penis to be curved ventrally.

Penile hypospadias is a more exaggerated form of hypospadias where the urethra opens on to the ventral surface of the penile shaft. Hypospadias should be repaired between the ages of four and five, to ensure both a good result and that the child, before starting school, no longer requires to sit down to pass urine. *Circumcision must not be permitted* as the prepuce is required for the repair. If the testicles are impalpable, full investigation of the sex must be undertaken in case the child is a **female pseudohermaphrodite**.

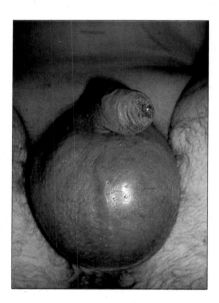

37.3 Urethral rupture. The history of a straddling injury to the perineum and the presence of extensive scrotal and perineal bruising with fresh blood oozing from the tip of the penis are sufficient for a diagnosis of membranous urethral trauma. Conservative management of the injury or primary repair may be undertaken, depending on the degree of injury as confirmed by a careful **ascending urethrogram**.

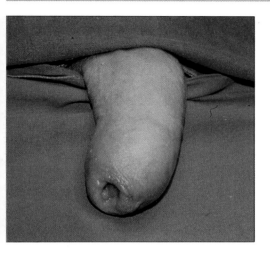

37.4 Phimosis. The foreskin is normally non-retractable during the first few months of life but, by the end of the first year, 50% will retract. It may be three to four years before all will do so. Should the foreskin remain non-retractile after the age of four, or there is evidence of recurrent balanitis, the prepuce can either be removed by circumcision, or adhesions between foreskin and glans divided before the prepuce is stretched.

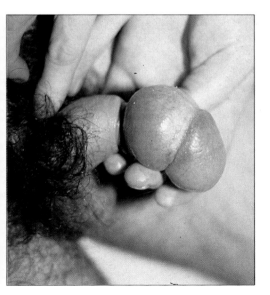

37.5 Paraphimosis. A poorly retracting foreskin, if it remains retracted, can act as a tight band and cause engorgement of the glans. Not infrequently, this may occur during early attempts at masturbation or sexual intercourse. It demands urgent treatment by compression of the glans and drawing the foreskin forwards, but if this fails, the tight band must be incised by dorsal slit, under general anaesthesia.

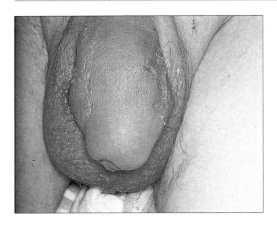

37.6 Peri-urethral abscess. The swollen, painful, tender and inflamed penis is due to a persistent urethritis which was neglected by the patient until the abscess developed.

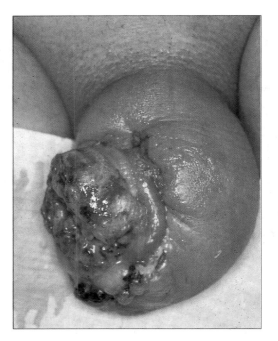

37.7 Carcinoma of the penis. This patient presented with a bloodstained purulent discharge from an advanced, ulcerating, squamous cell carcinoma with early lymphatic spread to inguinal lymph nodes. It is generally attributed to poor hygiene, associated with a non-retractable foreskin and only occurs in elderly patients. Early tumours respond dramatically to bleomycin, otherwise partial amputation and bilateral block dissection of inguinal lymph nodes may be required.

38.

TESTIS

Testicular and Spermatic Cord Anatomy

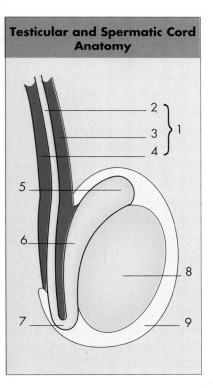

38.1 Diagrammatic representation of the testicle. The testicle has two component parts: the orchid which contains seminiferous tubules, and the epididymis, consisting of head, body and tail. The spermatic cord, containing the testicular vessels and vas, enters the head of the gland.

1 Spermatic cord
2 Vas deferens
3 Testicular artery
4 Pampiniform plexus of veins
5 Head of epididymis
6 Body of epididymis
7 Tail of epididymis
8 Orchid
9 Tunica vaginalis

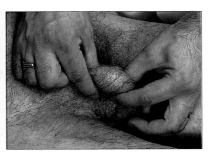

38.2 Clinical examination of the testicles. Scrotal examination is an integral part of the general examination. The cord structures are gently examined between finger and thumb of the examining hand and the testicle gently palpated for its component parts to determine its orientation. Transillumination of the scrotum is useful to determine whether enlargement is due to a cystic swelling.

303

Principle Differential Diagnosis of a Scrotal Swelling

- Hydrocele.
- Epididymal cyst/spermatocele.
- Epididymitis/orchitis.
- Torsion.
- Haematocele.
- Varicocele.
- Testicular tumour.
- Inguinal hernia.

Diagnosis

- General examination.
- Clinical examination of both testicles, spermatic cords and inguinal canals.
- Tumour markers (human gonadotrophin [beta-HCG], alphafetoprotein).
- Testicular ultrasonography.
- Chest radiograph.
- CT scanning.
- Lymphangiography.

MALDESCENT OF THE TESTIS

The testis can arrest in its descent to the scrotum within the inguinal canal, and, more rarely, within the abdomen. The testis is always smaller in size than normal. Both testes should be in the scrotum within 6 months of birth but excessively mobile or highly retractile testes commonly lie at the superficial inguinal ring. Where the testicle arrests in an ectopic position, the testicle is of normal size but does not lie in the line of descent and commonly remains in the superficial inguinal pouch or is transposed to perineal, femoral or prepubic sites. Maldescent of the testis is associated with an increased risk of neoplasia: 1 in 40 develop malignancy, rising to 1 in 20 if the testis remains within the abdomen.

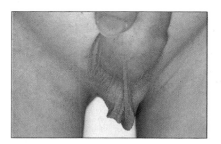

38.3 Incomplete testicular descent. Early operative placement of the testicle in a dartos pouch in the scrotum (orchidopexy) is essential to allow normal testicular development, preferably before the age of three years. Indirect inguinal hernias are frequently associated with the incomplete descent.

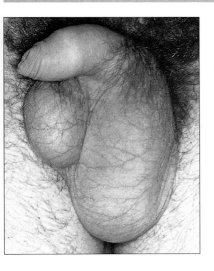

38.4 Hydrocele. This is a common condition particularly affecting older men. Serous fluid accumulates around the tunica albuginea resulting in painless scrotal enlargement. Most hydroceles are primary but they may be secondary to orchitis, torsion or, rarely, to a malignancy. The diagnosis is confirmed by transillumination. The swelling is smooth, the normal testis cannot be palpated and one can get above the swelling which differentiates it from an inguinal hernia. Hydoceles can be managed by aspiration, or by excision or inversion of the hydrocele sac.

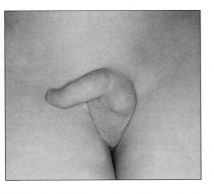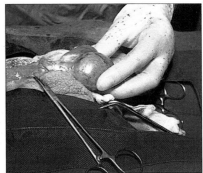

38.5 Testicular torsion. The patient is usually a teenager who presents with an acutely tender, swollen testis lying high within the scrotum, with an abnormal orientation (**left**). There may be a history of minor trauma and previous episodes of pain due to partial torsion. Exploration of the scrotum is mandatory and should occur as soon as possible as epididymo–orchitis is rare in this age group. At operation a 360° torsion was found with associated testicular infarction (**right**).

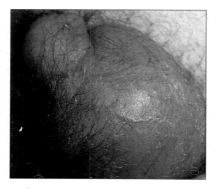

38.6 Epididymo–orchitis. Pain is severe but of a gradual onset, throbbing, and exacerbated by movement. The scrotum is red, tender and swollen. The testicle is exquisitely tender. Dysuria and frequency may be indicative of a concomitant urinary tract infection, confirmed by urine microscopy and culture. If both testes are involved, mumps should be suspected. Treatment consists of antibiotics if bacterial in origin, bed rest and scrotal support. Usual organisms are *Chlamydia* in younger men and coliforms in the older population.

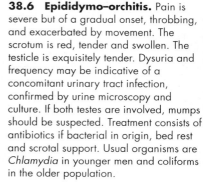

38.7 Epididymal cyst. The principle **differential diagnosis** is that of a hydrocele and varicele. Epididymal cysts are often multiple and lie above, behind and distinct from the testis. Surgery is not mandatory as most cysts are asymptomatic, and there is risk of damage to the pathway for spermatozoa.

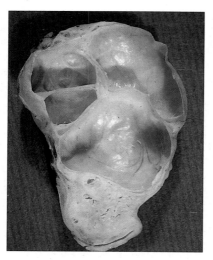

VARICOCELE

Dilatation of the pampiniform plexus of spermatic cord veins produces scrotal enlargement which resembles a bag of worms. It is more common on the left side because of the right-angle drainage of the testicular vein into the renal vein. It may be associated with infertility and a dragging sensation in the scrotum. Treatment is by transvenous embolisation or venous ligation at the level of the deep inguinal ring.

TESTICULAR TUMOURS

Tumours of the testis occur mainly in young men between 20 and 40 years of age. The principal types are **seminomas** and **teratomas**, which account for 90 per cent of all testicular tumours. Malignant lymphoma, yolk sac tumours, interstitial cell tumours and Sertoli/mesenchyme cell tumours make up the remainder. **Treatment** is primarily surgical with removal of the testicle through the inguinal canal. Initially, the spermatic cord is clamped to prevent tumour dissemination. Orchidectomy may be combined with a course of chemotherapy or radiotherapy depending on the histology and stage of the disease. Seminomas are particularly radio-sensitive, whereas teratomas are chemo-sensitive. The five-year survival rate for seminoma is 90–95 per cent and for early teratomas as high as 95 per cent.

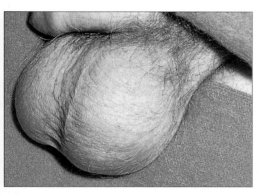

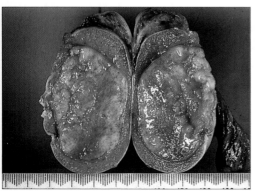

38.8 Seminoma. This 35-year-old patient presented with painless enlargement of his right testicle (***top***). He attributed this to a history of trauma which is common but misleading in such patients. The peak age for seminoma is between 30 and 40 years. The diagnosis is confirmed by elevated human chorionic gonadotrophin and alphafetoprotein. Metastases occur mainly via the lymphatics and may spread to the lungs. By comparison to teratomas, the cut surface of a seminoma has a rather amorphous, pale appearance (***bottom***).

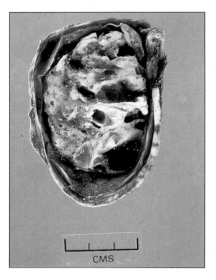

38.9 Teratoma. This lesion arises from primitive germinal cells and thus may contain cartilage, bone, muscle, fat and other tissues according to the degree of differentiation. Its peak age incidence is in the 20–30 years age-group. In 10% of cases the tumour may be bilateral.

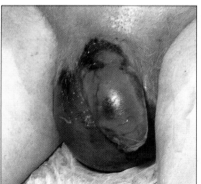

38.10 Fournier's gangrene of the scrotum. This is a necrotising fasciitis primarily affecting the subcutaneous fat and deep fascia of the perineum and scrotum due to blood-borne *haemolytic Streptococcus*. There is a cellulitis initially, associated with the appearance of dusky purple patches which progress to skin necrosis and crepitus. Treatment is by aggressive surgical debridement, intravenous antibiotics and cardiovascular support, but there is a substantial mortality.

Section 9

Neurology

39.

BRAIN AND MENINGES

RAISED INTRACRANIAL PRESSURE

The **cardinal symptoms and signs** associated with raised intracranial pressure are: headache, nausea, vomiting, visual disturbance, papiloedema, focal signs related to aetiological lesion; weight loss and anorexia may be present and usually indicate the presence of a tumour; bradycardia and mild hypertension are common in the later stages; intellectual deterioration and disorders of consciousness occur as intracranial pressure rises progressively; and enlargement of the head may be found in children prior to closure of the sutures.

Principal Differential Diagnosis
- Cerebral oedema (traumatic, infective).
- Space-occupying lesion (neoplasm, abscess, haematoma).
- Hydrocephalus.
- Post-meningitic.

Diagnosis
- General examination, including fundoscopy.
- Neurological examination of central and peripheral nervous system.
- Full blood count, serum biochemistry and viral titres where appropriate.
- Lumbar puncture and cerebro-spinal fluid (CSF) examination.
- Plain radiography of skull or spine.
- Chest radiograph (malignant disease).
- CT scanning.
- Magnetic resonance (MR) imaging.
- Angiography.
- Myelography.

COMA SCALE		
eyes open	spontaneously	4
	to speech	3
	to pain	2
	none	1
best verbal response	orientated	5
	confused	4
	inappropriate words	3
	incomprehensible sounds	2
	none	1
best motor response	obey commands	6
	purposeful movement	5
	withdrawal	4
	flexion to pain	3
	extension to pain	2
	none	1

39.1 Glasgow Coma Scale. Assessment of the level of consciousness is invaluable in the observation of patients with a variety of neurological disorders, when even minor changes in conscious level may indicate the need for urgent treatment. Although there are several coma classifications, the most widely adopted and useful is the Glasgow Coma Scale (GCS) which records the patient's responses to stimulation in terms of best eye opening responce, vocal response and motor response. It is particularly useful as trends in these parameters can be charted over time. Swelling, ischaemia or displacement of brain stem structures result in dysfunction of the reticular activating system in the brain stem which is concerned with consciousness. Brain stem compression, if untreated, leads to deterioration of conscious level, coma and death.

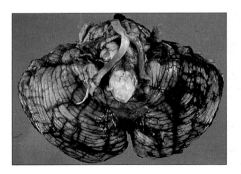

39.2   Pathological specimen indicating the effects of raised intracranial pressure. Death from raised intracranial pressure results from herniation of constituent parts of the brain through naturally occurring structures. Herniation may be transfalcine, where the cingulate gyrus hernia is beneath the free edge of falx; transtentorial, where the medial part of the temporal lobe is pushed downwards through the tentorial notch to become wedged between the tentorial edge and the mid-brain; and foraminal, where the cerebellar tonsils are displaced downwards through the foramen magnum, resulting in brainstem compression and death, as shown in this patient.

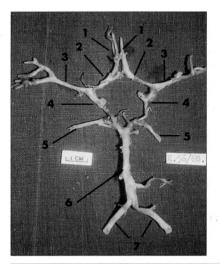

39.3   Circle of Willis. Aneurysms of the major intracranial blood vessels are relatively rare but the rupture accounts for a third of cerebral vascular accidents in patients less than 60 years of age. Haemorrhage from aneurysms is rare before the age of 20, with a sharp rise in incidence between 40 and 60, falling off rapidly thereafter. The aneurysms are usually sacular and are found at the major branches of the circle of Willis. Over 90% originate in the anterior part of the circle of Willis, the most common site being the internal carotid artery.

1	Anterior cerebral artery	5	Posterior cerebral artery
2	Anterior communicating artery	6	Basilar artery
3	Middle cerebral artery	7	Vertebral artery
4	Posterior communicating artery		

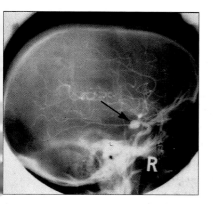

39.4 Berry aneurysm
(angiogram). Aneurysms are often single, but 10% of patients will have multiple aneurysms. Mirror image aneurysms are particularly common in the middle cerebral artery territory, where one in three will be so affected. For this reason alone, four-vessel angiography must be performed in all cases of subarachnoid haemorrhage. In this patient the aneurysm arises from the posterior communicating artery.

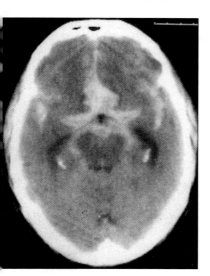

39.5 Subarachnoid haemorrhage
(CT scan). Small aneurysms are often unsuspected before the presenting sub-arachnoid haemorrhage. The rupture of an aneurysm may vary from a mild leakage of blood to a more major event with associated haematoma; survival will depend on the severity of this event. In this patient, blood fills the basal cisterns and outlines the brain stem. Overall, 10% of patients who have had a subarachnoid haemorrhage due to a ruptured berry aneurysm will be dead before their admission to hospital. The **overall mortality** due to this first bleed is 40%. Of those who survive the first haemorrhage without treatment, a third will be dead within a year from recurrent haemorrhage. This figure rises to two-thirds with the second haemorrhage and 80% with the third haemorrhage. Treatment may be either surgical or radiological intervention to obliterate the aneurysm.

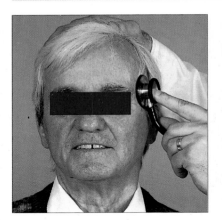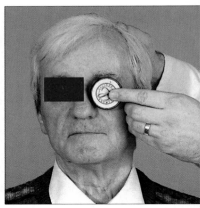

39.6 Auscultation of arterio–venous malformations. Symptoms arising from the patient's history and examination may suggest a cerebral aetiology for their presentation and the diagnosis of a suspected arterio–venous malformation can be made clinically by application of the stethoscope to either the temporal (***left***), frontal or occular (***right***) areas to detect the presence of a bruit.

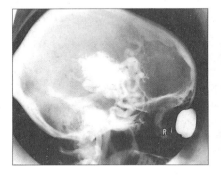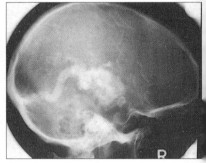

39.7 Arterio–venous malformation. A definitive diagnosis and a map of the feeding vessels is obtained by cerebral angiography, shown in the arterial (***left***) and venous (***right***) phases. This is essential in planning operative or radiological intervention to obliterate the feeding vessels. Untreated, there is the risk of catastrophic subarachnoid or intracerebral haemorrhage. Within ten years, 20% of patients will die and a further 30% will suffer severe disability from recurrent haemorrhage without treatment, which consists of surgical endovascular obliteration or radiosurgery (the 'gamma knife').

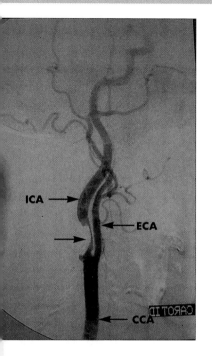

ICA →

← ECA

→

← CCA

39.8 Carotid artery stenosis.
Carotid artery disease is estimated to account for 50% of ischaemic cerebro-vascular accidents. Carotid artery disease most commonly affects the common carotid bifurcation and the proximal 2 cm of the internal carotid artery, as shown in this angiogram. Stroke may be caused by a haemodynamic obstruction to flow or, more commonly, by embolisation of plaque to the brain. Lesser degrees of injury lead to transient ischaemic attack (TIA, a stroke lasting less than 24 hours with complete recovery) and amaurosis fugax (transient loss of vision due to embolic occlusion of the central artery of the retina). Two large, multi-centre, randomised controlled trials have indicated that surgical removal of plaque (carotid endarterectomy) is significantly better than the best medical treatment at preventing stroke following TIA or amaurosis when the plaque causes 70% or greater narrowing of the artery. ICA=internal carotid artery; ECA=external carotid artery; CCA=common carotid artery.

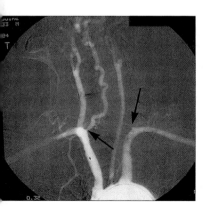

39.9 Vertebral artery stenosis. The
natural history of vertebral artery stenosis is poorly understood. This patient presented with vertebro–basilar insufficiency, and angiography demonstrated left vertebral occlusion and right vertebral artery origin stenosis. The patient underwent right vertebral artery endarterectomy with improvement in symptoms.

INTRACRANIAL NEOPLASMS

There is a **double peak age incidence** of intracranial neoplasms, with a small peak at 6–7 years of age, a decline in incidence until puberty and, thereafter, a progressive rise, with maximum incidence occurring in the fifth decade. As a rule they rarely metastasise and death usually results from the consequences of raised intracranial pressure and local pressure effects. The most common intracranial tumours are metastases, frequently from the lung and breast.

Classification

Skull

- Osteoma.
- Chordoma.
- Glomus jugulare tumour.
- Histiocytosis.
- Multiple myeloma.
- Paget's disease.
- Metastatic tumour.

Meninges

- Meningioma.

Pituitary and Parapituitary

- Chromophobe adenoma.
- Eosinophilic adenoma.
- Prolactinoma.
- Basophilic adenoma.
- Cranial pharyngioma.
- Cholesteatoma and neurinoma.

Intracerebral

- Metastases.
- Glioma.
- Ependymoma.
- Medulloblastoma.

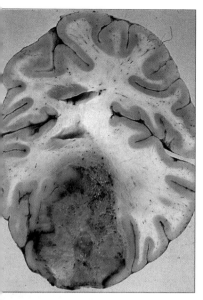

39.10 Pathological coronal section of glioma.

These are the most common primary tumours and account for 25% of intracranial tumours. Astrogliomas are initially slow-growing but may be rapidly invasive (glioblastoma multiforma), as in this patient. A less common form is an oligodendroglioma, which is slow-growing, sometimes calcified, and has less tendency to infiltrate the brain. There is a wide spectrum of tumour behaviour. Surgery, radiotherapy and steroids can all be useful.

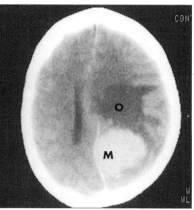

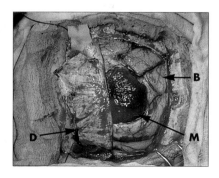

39.11   Meningioma. The CT scan shows a parasagittal meningioma (M) with associated oedema (O) anterior to the tumour (*left*). At operation the meningioma which was involving the sagittal sinus was exposed by reflecting the dura (D) to the left, and resected with part of the sinus (*right*). Meningiomas account for 20% of brain tumours and are slow-growing. They are usually found in close association with the dura which surrounds the brain (B).

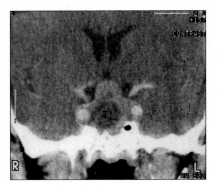

39.12 Pituitary tumour (coronal CT scan). This shows a large cystic tumour (T) with superior extension giving a 'cottage loaf' appearance. These lesions account for 15% of intracranial tumours and produce two types of symptoms: those related to local pressure, e.g. compression of the optic chiasm causing visual impairment and destruction of normal pituitary tissue causing symptoms of pituitary failure; and those due to the effects of hormonal hypersecretion.

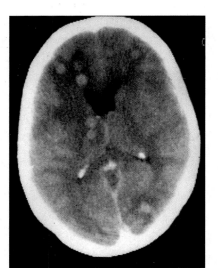

39.13 Metastatic tumour (CT scan). Multiple lesions seen on a CT scan in a patient presenting with symptoms of raised intracranial pressure. Multiple metastases, such as these, are inoperable and best treated with cytotoxic therapy, radiotherapy or hormonal manipulation if appropriate, with reduction of oedema by high-dose steroids such as dexa-methasone. If there is a solitary metastasis which is accessible, with no progression of primary tumour, then resection may be undertaken with an improvement in the quality of survival.

40.

HEAD INJURIES

It is important that head injuries, like trauma affecting organs elsewhere, should not be regarded in isolation. Particular attention is given to the mechanism of injury and, during the diagnostic and investigative phase of the acute injury, consideration is given to the **ABCs**: maintenance of **airway**, **breathing** and support for the **circulation,** if necessary.

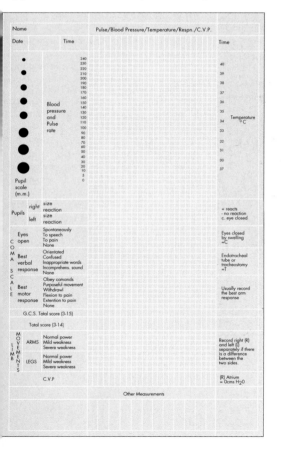

40.1 Head injury chart. Sequential observation of conscious level using the Glasgow Coma Scale, blood pressure and pulse and pupillary size provides information on the patient's wellbeing. The patient may or may not require admission to hospital, even if the head injury is of a simple nature. Many head injuries are alcohol related, due either to intoxication and collapse, or to impairment of senses and a resultant accident.

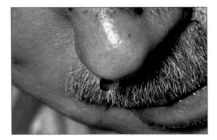

40.2 CSF rhinorrhoea. This patient sustained blunt head trauma following an assault. CSF rhinorrhoea is indicative of a base-of-skull fracture and, in this patient, involves the frontal sinus.

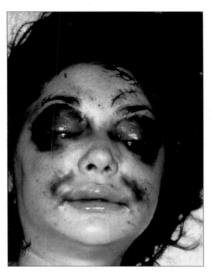

40.3 Anterior cranial fossa fracture. This type of fracture is indicated clinically (**top**) by the presence of periorbital haematomas, nasal bleeding, and nerve palsies affecting the first to fourth cranial nerves. Skull radiographs may or may not show the fracture. In this patient there is an 'H' type fracture (**bottom**). If fractures are compound, infection may occur in 5–10% of cases. Particular attention should be paid to the state of tetanus immunisation and the use of prophylactic antibiotics.

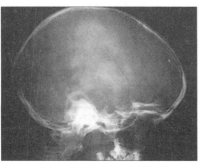

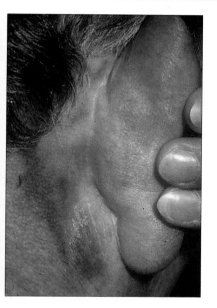

40.4 Middle cranial fossa fracture. This may be suspected clinically in this man fallen from his bicycle by bloody discharge from the ear and a mastoid haematoma (**Battle's sign**). Cranial nerve palsies affecting the seventh and eighth nerves may also be associated with this injury. One of the most common **preventable causes** of head injury seen in hospital Accident and Emergency departments is a fall from a bicycle. Widespread usage of cycle helmets to minimise head trauma would significantly reduce the incidence of serious head injury occurring in these accidents.

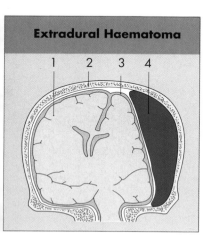

Extradural Haematoma

40.5 Diagrammatic representation of an extradural haematoma. This is an extradural collection of blood which may develop from a laceration of one or other of the meningeal vessels or venous sinuses, oozing from the diploe and bone on each side of the associated fracture.

1 Brain
2 Skull
3 Dura
4 Extradural haematoma

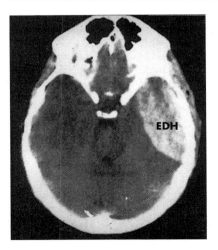

40.6 Extradural haematoma (CT scan). The skull fracture line crossed the middle meningeal artery which has resulted in this patient's extradural haematoma (EDH). The CT scan localises the clot accurately and helps plan the surgical evacuation.

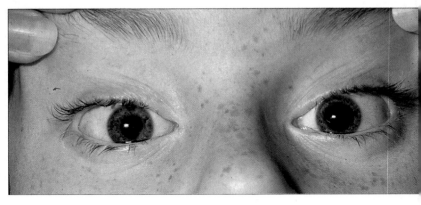

40.7 Fixed dilated pupil secondary to an expanding intracranial haematoma. This patient received a blow to the head from a cricket bat and was rendered unconscious for a few minutes and then apparently recovered. Two hours later he became confused and rapidly lost consciousness. This is one of the few neurosurgical emergencies where time is critical. If a CT scan is not available and the patient's condition is deteriorating, then the site to be explored may be suggested by the side on which there is a dilated pupil. The third cranial nerve becomes compressed on the ipsilateral side and there may be an associated scalp haematoma which overlies the extradural clot, because some of the extradural blood escapes through the fracture line to subcutaneous tissue, or simply because there is swelling at the site of injury.

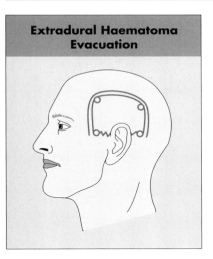

**Extradural Haematoma
Evacuation**

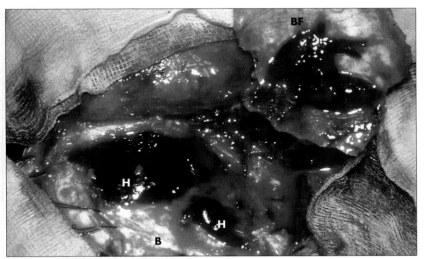

40.8 Evacuation of an extradural haematoma. Initially, a burr hole is created to evacuate the clot, then a craniotomy flap is raised (***top***) to identify the source of bleeding which is either ligated, clipped or diathermied. The operative illustration shows the bone flap (BF) raised superiorly and to the left, with some clot adhering to its undersurface and residual clot lying on the dura (***bottom***). If surgery is done early enough, the outlook is excellent. B = brain; H = haematoma.

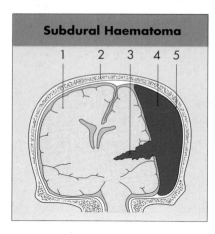

Subdural Haematoma

1 2 3 4 5

40.9 Diagrammatic representation of subdural haematoma. This results from bleeding into the subdural space from lacerated or pulped cerebrum, and is usually part of an overwhelming head injury. The patient frequently presents in deep coma from the moment of injury, with further deterioration.

1 Brain
2 Skull
3 Laceration of the brain
4 Subdural haematoma
5 Dura

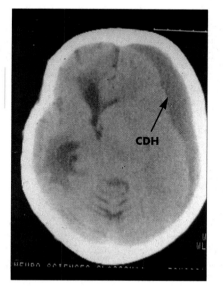

CDH

40.10 Chronic subdural haematoma (CDH) (CT scan). The haematoma has caused midline shift. This occurs from a trivial injury sustained weeks prior to admission. Usually a small tear in the cerebral vein occurs as it traverses the subdural space. With raised venous pressure when the patient coughs, strains or bends over, a little blood extravasates, resulting in a haematoma which becomes encapsulated. There may be some degree of blood breakdown, giving rise to a hygroma which exerts its own osmotic pressure, drawing more fluid in, and so enlarging. Clinical features are those of progressive mental deterioration, headaches, vomiting, drowsiness and coma. In half the patients, these lesions can be bilateral. Treatment is by way of drainage through burr holes, and the prognosis is good.

41.

SPINAL CORD

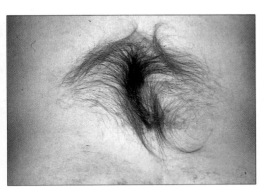

41.1 Spina bifida occulta. The isolated tuft of hair on the back at the base of the spine is indicative of an underlying spina bifida occulta. Radiographs may reveal an abnormality of the lamina or failure of fusion of the laminar arch. It may be asymptomatic, but fibrous bands tethering the cord may produce paraesthesia or sphincter disorders.

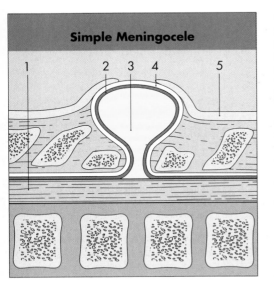

Simple Meningocele

41.2 Diagrammatic representation of a simple meningocele. This defect can occur anywhere in the spine, but usually occurs in the lumbar region and results from failure of fusion of the lamina. The subarachnoid space protrudes through the defect and the arachnoid membrane fuses with the skin to which the nerve roots may be adherent.

1 Spinal cord and roots
2 Meninges
3 CSF-filled sac
4 Skin defect
5 Skin

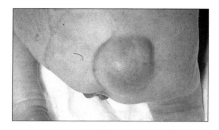

41.3 Lumbar meningocele. The cord is normal and usually there are no neurological abnormalities. These lesions can be detected by antenatal ultrasonography.

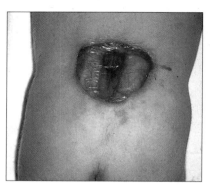

41.4 Lumbar myelomeningocele. Myelomeningocele is a much more severe defect where the spinal nerve roots and spinal cord adhere to the membrane, resulting in exposure of neural tissue and leakage of CSF. The neonate is at high risk of meningitis and hydrocephalus, and there is usually both sensory and motor loss affecting the lower limbs and sphincters. Major spina bifida defects such as this can be detected prenatally by alphafetoprotein rises in the maternal blood.

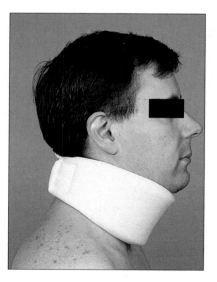

41.5 Whiplash injury to cervical spine. This patient is wearing a soft cervical collar as part of the management of a forced extension injury to the cervical spine following a head-on collision with another vehicle. The plain radiographs showed straightening of the cervical spine indicative of muscular spasm following trauma. It is vital that all seven cervical vertebrae are seen, even with the aid of a transaxillary view of the cervico–thoracic junction (swimmer's view). There was no fracture and the patient regained full neck movement after taking non-steroidal anti-inflammatory drugs for five days.

Whiplash injuries of this nature, although still potentially serious, have been reduced to a great extent by the compulsory fitting of head restraints in motor vehicles. This prevents the full forced extension injury.

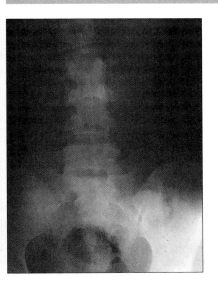

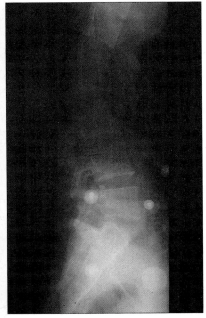

41.6 Angulated displaced fracture of the lumbar spine.

The importance of two radiographic views is emphasised by this particular type of fracture where, in the antero–posterior view (***top***), there appears to be minimal trauma to the spine but, on the lateral (***bottom***) view, there is severe displacement and angulation secondary to a forced flexion injury with restraint from a seat belt. Surprisingly, this patient did not have any signs of cord compression. Correction was undertaken by straightening of the spine and stabilisation using internal fixation.

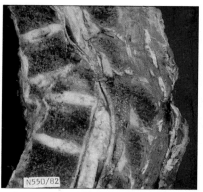

41.7 Pathological specimens of traumatic spinal cord compression.
These examples occurred following major road traffic accident trauma. In the first patient, a hyperflexion injury has transected the cord (***top***); in the second, a fracture dislocation has resulted in severe cord compression (***middle***); and in the third, the patient survived for five weeks following trauma to the mid-thoracic cord and succumbed from multi-organ failure due to associated injuries (***bottom***).

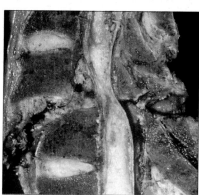

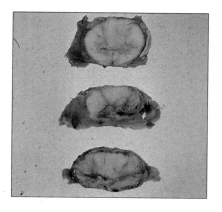

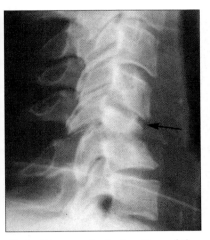 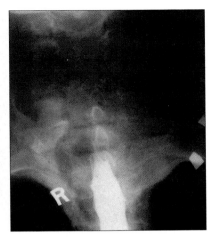

41.8 Metastatic destruction of the cervical vertebral body. After minor trauma, this patient presented with sudden- onset quadriplegia due to the collapse, angulation and displacement of a cervical vertebral body (***left***). Although CT or MR imaging is preferable to delineate the injury, myelography, as shown, is often used out of hours (***right***).

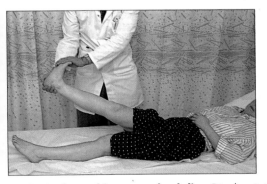

41.9 Prolapsed intervertebral disc. Disc herniation results in protrusion of the nucleus pulposus, most commonly postero–laterally or directly posteriorly through a defect in the nucleus pulposus. It is usually initiated by trauma and principally affects active adult males, the most common sites being between L_4/L_5 and L_5/S_1. Most patients complain of sciatic pain which is unilateral, radiating from the buttock along the back of the thigh and knee to the lateral side of the foot, and which is aggravated by raising the intra-thecal pressure by coughing, sneezing or straining, or by straight-leg raising as shown here, which stretches the sciatic nerve.

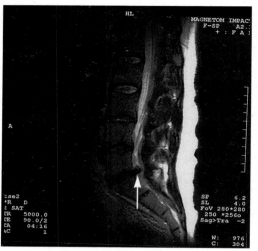

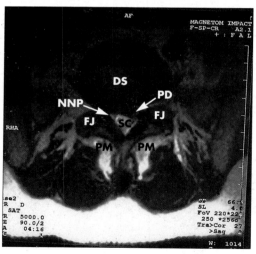

41.10 Prolapsed intervertebral disc (MR scan). This investigation confirms the diagnosis showing, in this patient, clear extrinsic compression of the spinal nerve root in the sagittal plane (***top***) and in the axial plane (***bottom***). Clinically, the **differential diagnosis** includes sacro–ileitis, osteoarthritis, spondylolisthesis, spinal tumour, tuberculosis, intra-pelvic tumour (prostate, rectum) involving the sacral plexus, and intermittent claudication. Most patients with a prolapsed disc settle conservatively, but some require radiological (chymopapain intra-disc injection leading to nucleolysis) or surgical intervention.

42.

PERIPHERAL NERVE INJURIES

Following injury to the peripheral nerves, recovery by regrowth of axons depends on the degree of injury and the severity of trauma. The resultant neurological deficit, if any, will depend on the type of nerve and the respective loss of its sensory and/or motor components. **Neuropraxia** is damage to the nerve fibres without loss of continuity of the axis cylinder. The conduction along the fibres is interrupted only for a short period of time and recovery is usually complete within a few days. **Axonotmesis** is an injury to the axon without disruption of the continuity of its sheath. The axon undergoes Wallerian degeneration and recovery requires that the axons regenerate and grow down into the intact sheath. The rate of regeneration is approximately 3–4 mm a day and therefore the more proximal the injury, the longer it will be before full functional recovery occurs. Excessive fibrosis may hinder growth so that reinnervation is delayed and the final functional result is less than perfect.

Brachial plexus injuries may be associated with severe trauma during either a road traffic accident or an obstetric delivery. Lesser degrees of trauma to the brachial plexus may be inflicted following attempted subclavian line insertion with or without resultant haematoma. Injury to the brachial plexus is usually transient and full recovery is the norm.

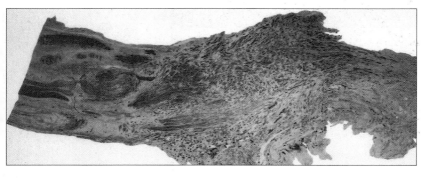

42.1   Neuroma secondary to neurotmesis. Neurotmesis is physical disruption of the peripheral nerve. Fibrous tissue forms between the divided nerve ends and, although the divided axons attempt to grow distally (at the rate of 1 mm per day), reinnervation of end organs is unusual.

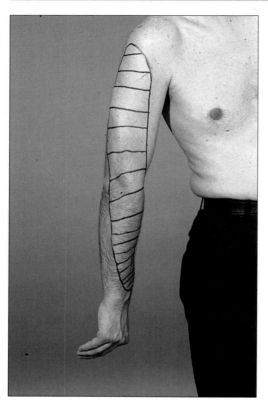

42.2 Upper lesion (Erb's palsy). There is damage to C_5/C_6, with resultant paralysis of the biceps, brachialis, brachioradialis, supinator and deltoid. The resultant deficit causes the arm to be internally rotated and the forearm pronated, and gives impaired sensation of the outer side of the upper arm.

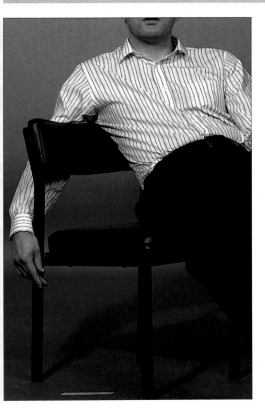

42.3 Mechanism of radial nerve injury. A neuropraxic-type injury will result from compression of the radial nerve against the spiral groove on the humerus. This is not an uncommon injury in patients who are inebriated. Alternatively, a fracture of the shaft of the humerus may result in radial nerve injury.

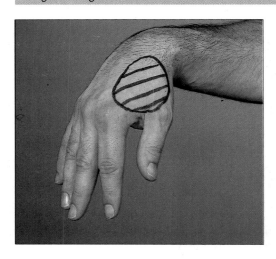

42.4 Radial nerve injury.
The resultant deficit causes wrist drop due to paralysis of the wrist extensors and impaired sensation over a small area of the dorsum of the hand at the base of the index finger and thumb.

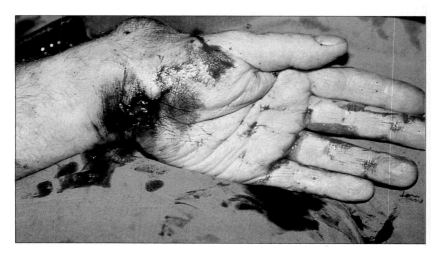

42.5 Mechanism of median nerve injury. This patient suffered a severe compound distal radius and ulnar fracture resulting in an axonotmesis-type injury. More commonly, median nerve injuries are due to penetrating wounds resulting from knife injuries or glass shards. Lacerations around the wrist joint must be explored, not only for neural injury but associated tendon and vascular injury.

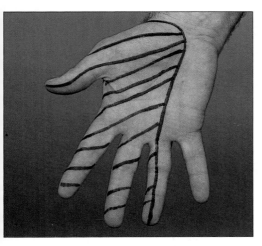

42.6 Median nerve injury. Injury at the wrist causes thenar wasting and diminished sensation in the radial three-and-a-half digits (*top*). Loss of power in the thenar muscles results in a monkey-grip with the patient being unable to oppose the thumb to the other four digits (*bottom*).

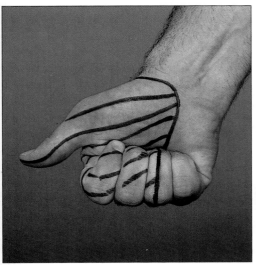

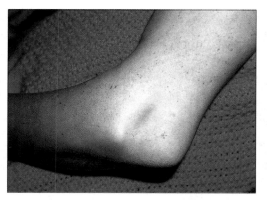

42.7 Mechanism of ulnar nerve injury. Like other peripheral nerves, the ulnar nerve is susceptible to injury by external penetration or by fracture trauma from within. In this patient a neuropraxia occurred due to dislocation of the elbow (***top***) which was confirmed radiologically (***bottom***).

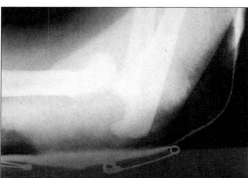

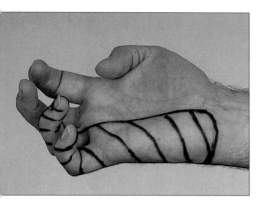

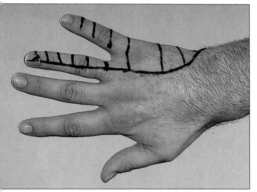

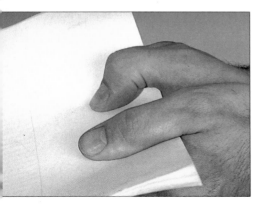

42.8 Ulnar nerve injury. This produces the typical deformity of a clawed-hand or 'main-en-griffe' (***top***). The clawed appearance results from an opposed action of the long flexors and extensors of the fingers. There is also impaired sensation of the ulnar one-and-a-half digits and the ulnar border of the hand (***middle***). Froment's sign results because of paralysis of the adductor pollicis, so that if a patient holds a piece of paper between the index finger and thumb, the thumb flexes in the affected right hand (***bottom***).

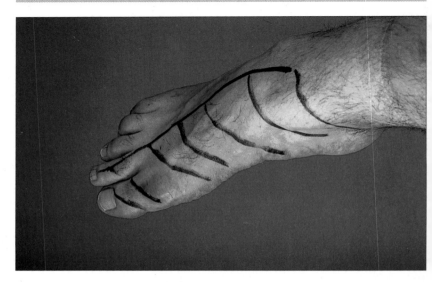

42.9 Common peroneal nerve injury. This nerve is at particular risk as it winds round the neck of the fibula. It may be injured in association with a fractured neck of the fibula, because a plaster of paris cast is applied too tightly, or as a result of misplaced enthusiasm when performing multiple stab avulsions of varicose veins. The **resultant deficit** causes foot drop due to paralysis of the ankle and foot extensors, and inversion of the foot due to paralysis of the peroneal muscles with an unopposed action of the foot flexors and invertors. There is impaired sensation over the medial side of the dorsum of the foot.

Index

Page references in bold type refer to illustrations.

ABC (airway, breathing and circulation), 319
abdomen, 115–230
  acute, 116–20
abdominal aortic aneurysm, 248–52
abscess
  abdominal, 119–20
  ano-rectal, **214**
  apical, **69**
  breast, 29, 30
  hepatic, **137**
    amoebic, **138**
  ischiorectal, **215**
  lung, 88
  perianal, **214**
  peri-urethral, **302**
  pyogenic, **137**
  subphrenic, 88, **120**
acanthosis nigrans, **57**
achalasia, 106, **106**
actinomycosis, 5
acute abdomen, 116–20
acute respiratory distress syndrome, **87**
adenocarcinoma, oesophagus, **109**
adenoid enlargement, **82**
adenoma
  adrenocortical, **279**
  follicular, thyroid, **271**
  hepatic, **143**
  parathyroid, **274**
  pleomorphic, parotid gland, **80**
  villous, colorectal, **205**
adhesive intestinal obstruction, **184, 185**
adnexae, 37–58
adrenal gland, 275–80
adrenal medullary tumours, 279–80
aldosteronism, primary, **275**
ameloblastoma, 75
amoebic liver abscess, **138**
amputation, below-knee, **245**
anal canal, 209–17
  anatomy, **209**
anal pain, differential diagnosis, 210
anal warts, **217**
anatomy
  anal canal, **209**
  arterial, lower limb, **240**
  bilary system, **147**
  femoral canal, **223**
  inguinal canal, **219**
  liver, **133**
  neck, **20**
  parotid gland, **78**
  spermatic cord, **303**
  testis, **303**
  thyroid, **266**

aneurysm
  aorta
    abdominal, 248–52
    dissecting, **102**
    thoracic, **247**
  arterial disease, 247–52
  Berry, **313**
  iliac artery, **251**
  popliteal artery, **252**
  splenic artery, **177**
angina pectoris, 97
angiodysplasia, colonoscopy, **202**
ankle pressures, Doppler ultrasound, **236**
ano-rectal abscess, **214**
anus
  fistula, **212**
  imperforate, **180**
  squamous cell carcinoma, **217**
aorta
  aneurysm
    abdominal, 248–52
    dissecting, **102**
    thoracic, **247**
  coarctation, **95**
  disease, 95–7
  occlusion, **238**
  stenosis, **96**
  traumatic dissection, **102**
aortic valve, **96**
aorto-caval fistula, **251**
aortography, thoracic, **248**
apical abscess, **69**
appendicitis, acute, 195
appendix, 194–6
  carcinoid, **196**
  mucocele, **196**
arcus senilis, **97**
ARDS (acute respiratory distress syndrome), 87
arm, ischaemia, 243–6
arterial anatomy, lower limb, **240**
arterial disease
  aneurysmal, 247–52
  occlusive, 232–46
arterio-venous malformation, **314**
aspiration pneumonia, 86
atelectasis, pulmonary, **17**
atherosclerosis, 99
atresia
  biliary, **149**
  duodenal, **122**
  ileal, **179**
  oesophageal, **104**
atrial myxoma, **97**
auscultation
  arterio-venous malformation, **314**
  Hunter's canal, **236**
axillary embolus, **244**

axillary nodes, **25**
axillary vein, spontaneous thrombosis, **262, 263**
axonotmesis, 331

Barrett's oesophagus, **107**
basal cell carcinoma, **51, 52**
bell sign, 113
below-knee amputation, **245**
benign pigmented moles, 48–50
benign prostatic hypertrophy, **298**
benign tumour, skin, 44–8
Berry aneurysm, **313**
bilary system, anatomy, **147**
bile ducts, 146–58
    injury, **156**
    see also choledochal
biliary atresia, **149**
biliary stricture, benign, **156**
biliary tree
    laparoscopic ultrasonography, **153**
    parasitic infestation, **155**
bladder, 295–7
    calculus, **296**
    carcinoma, **297**
    transitional cell carcinoma, **296**
blue naevus, **50**
body area percentages, **9**
Boerhaave's syndrome, 105
bowel, see large bowel; small bowel
Bowen's disease, **50**
brachial plexus injury, 331
brain, 310–18
branchial cyst, **23**
branchial fistula, **22, 23**
breast, 24–36
    abscess, **29**
        lactational, **30**
        non-lactational, **29**
    accessory tissue, **27**
    asymmetry, **26**
    cystic disease, **30, 31**
    lymphatic drainage, **25**
    pathology, frequency, **26**
    swelling, differential diagnosis, 24
breast carcinoma, **32**
    inflammatory, **34**
    mammography, **33**
    recurrent, **36**
    ulcerated, **34**
bronchial carcinoma, **90**
buccal mucosa, carcinoma, **71**
Buerger's disease, **246**
Buerger's sign, 237
bulla of the lung, **88**
burns, 9–12, **10–11**
bypass grafts, **240, 241**

caecum, volvulus, **186**
calculus
    bladder, **296**
    staghorn, **289**
    ureter, **289**
cancer, *see specific sites and types*
candidiasis, oesophageal, **107**
carcinoid flush, **58**

carcinoma, *see specific sites and types*
caries, **73**
carotid artery, stenosis, **315**
cellulitis, periorbital, **4**
central line, **13**
cerebrospinal fluid rhinorrhea, **320**
cervical spine, whiplash injury, **326**
chest deformity, **111**
chest wall, 86–91
    trauma, 91
cholangiocarcinoma, **158**
    percutaneous transhepatic biliary drainage, **157**
cholangiography, operative, **153**
cholangitis, **154**
cholecystitis, **151, 152**
choledochal cyst, **150**
choledocholithiasis, **154**
cholelithiasis, **150**
Chvostek's sign, **273**
chyluria, **294**
circle of Willis, **312**
cirrhosis, micronodular, **140**
clawed hand, 337
cleft lip, **68–9**
Clonorchis sinensis, 155
Clostridium tetani, 5
CLOtest, **124**
cold sore, **66**
colitis
    ischaemic, **202**
    pseudomembranous, **202**
    ulcerative, **200,** 200–3
        pathological specimen, **201**
colon, 197–208
    cancer, stages, 204
    carcinoma, 203, **207**
    polypoidal, **208**
colorectal hepatic metastasis, **145**
colorectal neoplasm, 203–8
colo-vesical fistula, **200**
coma scale, **311**
common bile duct, injury, **156**
compression bandaging, **259**
congenital heart disease, 92–5
Conn's syndrome, **275**
coronary artery, stenosis, **98**
Couvoisier's law, **168**
cranial fossa, fracture, **320, 321**
Crohn's disease, **190, 201**
crural disease, **241**
Cullen's sign, **162**
Cushing's syndrome, **277, 278**
cutaneous infections, acute, 2–4
cyanosis, 93
cyst, *see specific sites and types*
cystic hygroma, **22**
cystoadenoma, pancreas, **170**
cystogram, micturating, **286**
cytology, fine-needle aspirate, **119**

deep venous thrombosis, **16**, 260–4
    iliofemoral, **261**
dental cyst, **75**
dentigerous cyst, 75
dermatofibroma, **44**

rmoid cyst, **39**
phragmatic hernia, 110–14
  acquired, **112**
  congenital, 110–11
  traumatic, **114**
ferential diagnoses
  acute appendicitis, 195
  acute tonsillitis, 83
  anal pain, 210
  angiodysplasia, 202
  biliary atresia, 149
  breast swelling, 24
  dysphagia, 103
  epididymal cyst, 306
  groin swellings, 255
  gynaecology, surgical, 227
  hypertension, 99
  intervertebral disc prolapse, 330
  intestinal obstruction, 179
  intracranial pressure, raised, 310
  jaundice, obstructive, 148
  jaw cysts, 75
  keratoacanthoma, 45
  lip carcinoma, 67
  lymphadenopathy, 21
  mediastinal shadowing, 100
  neck swelling, 19, 20
  pancreatitis, acute, 161
  perforated terminal ileitis, **189**
  phaeochromocytoma, 280
  pneumoperitoneum, **127**
  polyarteritis nodosa, small bowel, **191**
  pruritus ani, 210
  pyloric stenosis, 122
  renal mass, 282
  scrotal swelling, 304
  splenomegaly, 173
  thyroglossal cyst, 23
  transitional cell carcinoma, bladder, 296
  ulcerative colitis, 200
  umbilical fistula, 187
  urine retention, chronic, 297
  Wilms' tumour, 291
diverticular disease, 199–200
diverticulitis, 199
diverticulosis, **189, 199**
dorsalis pedis artery, palpation, **235**
drug hypersensitivity rash, **16**
duodenitis, **123**
duodenum, 121–31
  atresia, **122**
  fistula, **18**
  ulcer, **123**
    bleeding, **124**
    chronic, **125**
Dupuytren's contracture, **40**
dysphagia, 103

early gastric cancer (EGC), **130**
ectopia vesicae, **295**
ectopic pregnancy, ruptured, **230**
eczema
  nipple, 24
  varicose, **257**
Eisenmenger syndrome, **93**
embolisation, distal, **243**

emphysema, surgical, **91**
empyema, **88**
endocrinology, 265–80
endoscopic retrograde
  cholangiopancreatography (ERCP), 146, 150,
    154, 155
epididymal cyst, **306**
epididymo-orchitis, **306**
epulis, **74**
Erb's palsy, **332**
eruption cyst, 75
erysipelas, **4**
erythema
  ab igne, 10
  necrolytic migratory, **172**
  nodosum, **190**
erythroplakia, oral cavity, **70**
eschar, **74**
exit site infection, **13**
extradural haematoma, **321, 322**
  evacuation, **323**

facial fractures, 60–3
facial nerve palsy, **80**
facial sinus, **74**
faecal occult blood, **118**
Fallot's tetralogy, **94**
familial adenomatous polyposis, **205**
fasciitis, necrotizing, **6–7**
fasciotomy, **243**
femoral artery
  palpation, **234**
  stenosis, **239, 240**
femoral canal, anatomy, **223**
femoral hernia, **224**
femoro-popliteal bypass graft, **240**
fibroadenoma, breast, **31, 32**
fibromuscular dysplasia, 99
fibronodular hyperplasia, **142**
fibrosarcoma, **52**
fimbrial cyst, torsion, **229**
fine-needle aspiration
  acute abdomen, **119**
  thyroid follicular carcinoma, **272**
finger clubbing, **57**
fistula
  in ano, **213**
  branchial, **22, 23**
  duodenal, **18**
  mammary duct, **30**
  pancreatic, **165**
flail chest, 91
floor of the mouth, carcinoma, **71**
follicular adenoma, thyroid, **271**
follicular carcinoma, thyroid, **272**
folliculitis, **3**
foot, ischaemic ulcer, **237**
foot drop, 338
foreign body, swallowed, **104**
Fournier's gangrene, scrotum, **308**
fracture
  cranial fossa, **320, 321**
  lumbar spine, **327**
fractures, facial, 60–3
frostbite, **245**
fungal infection, perineal, **8**

gallbladder, 146–58
  abnormalities, 149
  carcinoma, **155**
  mucocele, **152**
  ultrasonography, **151**
gallstone ileus, **192**
gangrene
  foot, **237**
  Fournier's, **308**
  gas, **6**
gastric erosions, acute, **125**
gastric polyposis, **127**
gastric resection, **131**
gastric ulcer, chronic, **125**
gastric varix, **141**
gastric volvulus, **127**
geographic tongue, **72**
giant hairy naevus, **49**
giant lipoma, **48**
Glasgow coma scale, **311**
glioma, **317**
glossitis, median rhomboid, **72**
glucagonoma, **172**
goitre, 267, **268**
Goodsall's rule, 212
Graves' disease, **270**
great vessels, 92–9
Grey Turner's sign, **162**
gums, 73–4
gynaecology, surgical, 227–30
gynaecomastia, **29**

haemangioma, **45, 46**
haematoma
  after femoral artery puncture, **17**
  extradural, **321, 322**
    evacuation, **323**
  intrahepatic, **136**
  subdural, **324**
  subungual, **42**
  wound, **14**
haemoccult test, **118**
haemorrhage, subarachnoid, **313**
haemorrhoids, **211**
  prolapsed thrombosed, **212**
hairy cell leukemia, spleen, **175**
hand
  clawed, **337**
  ischaemic, **245**
Hashimoto's thyroiditis, **269**
head injuries, 319–24
  chart, **319**
heartburn, 113
heart disease, 92–9
  congenital, 92–5
  cyanotic, **93**
  ischaemic, 97–8
Helicobacter pylori, CLOtest, **124**
Heller's operation, 106
hepatic abscess, **137, 138**
hepatic adenoma, **143**
hepatic cyst, **135**
hepatic metastasis
  colorectal, **145**
  from sigmoid tumour, **208**

hepatic trauma, **136**
hepatocellular carcinoma, **143**
hepatoma, **144, 145**
hepatomegaly, 132
hernia, 218–26
  diaphragmatic, 110–14, **112, 114**
  femoral, **224**
  hiatus, **113**
  incisional, **16, 226**
  inguinal, **221, 222, 223**
  inguino-scrotal, **222**
  internal, Meckel's diverticulum, **189**
  Lichtenstein repair, **221**
  obturator, **224**
  para-umbilical, **225**
  Richter's, **225**
  umbilical, **218**
herniation, disc, 329
herniogram, **220**
herpes simplex, **66**
herpes zoster, **58**
hiatus hernia, **113**
Hirschsprung's disease, **181**
Hunter's canal, auscultation, **236**
hydatid cyst, **138, 139**
hydradenitis suppurativa, **3**
hydrocele, testis, **305**
hydroureter, **287**
hygroma, cystic, **22**
hyperparathyroidism, primary, **274**
hypertension, 99
hyperthyroidism, 270
hypoadrenocorticism, 276–9
hypospadias, **299, 300**
hypothyroidism, 269

idiothrombocytopenic purpura, **176**
ileal atresia, **179**
ileitis, terminal, **189**
ileostomy, **203**
ileum, multiple diverticulosis, **189**
iliac artery
  aneurysm, **251**
  'kissing' stent placement, **239**
  stenosis, **238**
infection
  cutaneous, acute, 2–4
  exit site, **13**
  fungal, perineal, **8**
  oro-facial, **73**
  specific, 5–8
  wound, **14, 15**
inferior vena cava, anti-embolic filter, **262**
ingrowing toenail, **41**
inguinal canal, anatomy, **219**
inguinal hernia, **221, 222, 223**
  paediatric, **220**
inguino-scrotal hernia, **222**
insulinoma, **171**
intervertebral disc, prolapsed, **329, 330**
intracranial neoplasm, 316–18
intracranial pressure, raised
  differential diagnosis, 310
  pathological specimen, **312**
intracranial tumour, metastatic, **317**
intravenous urogram, **283**

tussusception, **182, 183**
chaemia
  hand, **245**
  limb, 233, 242–6
chaemic colitis, **202**

undice, 148, **148**
w, 73–4
  cysts, 75
ejunum, diverticulum, **187**
uvenile polyp, **183**

eloid scar, hypertrophic, **12**
eratoacanthoma, **45**
eratocyst, 75
eratosis, seborrhoeic, **44**
idney, 282–94
  palpation, **283**
  solitary, **284**
  stone formation, 288
  see also renal
Killian's dehiscence, 84
Klatskin tumour, 157, **158**

aparoscopic ultrasonography
  biliary tree, **153**
  pancreatic carcinoma, **169**
aparoscopy
  acute appendicitis, 195
  diagnostic, **119**
  inguinal hernia, **222**
  liver biopsy, **134**
  trans-cystic duct exploration, **153**
laparotomy, multiple, **184**
large bowel
  carcinoma, **206**
  lymphatic drainage, **198**
latissimus dorsi flap reconstruction, **35**
leg
  arterial anatomy, **240**
  venous drainage, **253**
leiomyoma
  gastric, **129**
  small bowel, **193**
leiomyosarcoma, fundus, **129**
lentigo maligna, **54**
leukoplakia, 64
  oral cavity, **70**
Lichtenstein repair, hernia, **221**
limb ischaemia, 233
  acute, 242–3
  chronic, 233, **237**
  upper, 243–6
linitis plastica, **131**
lipodermatosclerosis, **257**
lipoma, **47, 48**
lips, 66–7
  carcinoma, **68**
  see also cleft lip
liver, 132–45
  anatomy, segmental, **133**
  haematoma, **136**
  laparoscopic biopsy, **134**
  neoplasm, 142–3
  polycystic disease, **135**
  systemic disease signs, **133, 134**

  see also hepatic
lumbar spine, fracture, **327**
lung, 86–91
  abscess, 88
  bulla, **88**
  carcinoma, **89**
  tumour, 89–90
  see also pulmonary
lymphadenopathy, **21, 22**
lymphatic vessels, 253–64
  breast, **25**
  large bowel, **198**
lymphoedema, **36, 264**
lymphoma, small bowel, **193**

macrocheilia, **66**
main-en-griffe, 337
maldescent of the testis, 304, **304**
malignant disease, 24
  oral cavity, 64
  systemic, skin changes, 57–8
malignant melanoma, 53–6
  amelanotic, **54**
  metastatic, **56**
  nodular, **55**
  plantar acral, **56**
  subungual, **56**
  superficial spreading, **54**
Mallory-Weiss tear, **104**
mammary duct, fistula, **30**
mammography, carcinoma, **33**
mandible, fractured, **63**
manometry, oesophagus, **106**
Marjolin's ulcer, **50**, 259
mastitis, periductal, 28
maxillary antrum, carcinoma, **76**
Meckel's diverticulum, **187**
  and internal hernia, **189**
  symptomatic, **188**
median nerve, injury, **334, 335**
mediastinum, 100–1
megacolon, toxic, **201**
melanocytic naevus, **48**
melanoma, see malignant melanoma
meninges, 310–18
meningioma, **317**
meningocele
  lumbar, **326**
  simple, **325**
mesenteric infarction, **191**
mid-face, central fracture, **62**
mitral valve
  disease, 95–7
  stenosis, **96**
moles, benign pigmented, 48–50
mouth, see oral cavity
mucocele, gallbladder, **152**
Murphy's sign, 151
myelofibrosis, spleen, **174**
myelomeningocele, lumbar, **326**
myxoedema, **269**
myxoma, atrial, **97**

naevus
  blue, **50**
  giant hairy, **49**

melanocytic, **48**
strawberry, **46**
nasopharyngeal carcinoma, **83**
nasopharynx, 82
carcinoma, **83**
neck, 19–23
anatomy, **20**
differential diagnosis, 19, 20
swelling, 19–20
necrolytic migratory erythema, **172**
necrosis, peripancreatic, **164**
necrotizing fasciitis, **6–7**
neoplasm, *see specific sites and types*
nephroblastoma, **291**
nerves
peripheral, injuries, 331–8
upper lesion, **332**
neuroblastoma, **280**
neurofibroma, **47**
neurology, 309–38
neuroma, **331**
neuronal intestinal dysplasia, **181**
neuropraxia, 331
neurotmesis, 331
nipple
accessory, **26**
discharge, **29**
eczema, 24, **27**
inversion, **28**
nose, fractured, **60**

obstruction
intestinal, 178–86
adhesive, **184, 185**
differential diagnosis, 179
pelvi-ureteric junction, **286**
occlusion
femoro-popliteal, 239–40
infra-popliteal, 241–2
oesophagitis, **114**
oesophagus, 103–9
adenocarcinoma, **109**
atresia, **104**
candidiasis, **107**
manometry, **106**
neoplasm, 108
perforation, **105**
squamous cell carcinoma, **108**
varix, **141**
onychogryphosis, **42**
oral cavity, 64–76, **70–1**
malignant tumours, 76
mouth floor, carcinoma, **71**
oral thrush, **65**
orbital floor, fractured, **61, 62**
oro-facial infection, **73**
oromaxillofacial region, 59–84
oropharynx, 82
osteitis fibrosa cystica, fingers, **274**
osteogenic sarcoma, **76**
ovary
bleeding cyst, **229**
Kruckenberg tumour, **230**

Paget's disease, **27**
pain, abdomen, 116

localisation, **118**
palate, 66–7
cleft, **68–9**
pancreas, 159–72
annular, **160**
carcinoma, **169**
Couvoisier's law, **168**
Whipple's resection, **170**
cystadenoma, **170**
fistula, **165**
neoplasm, 161, 167
pseudocyst, **164, 165**
pancreas divisum, **160**
pancreatitis
acute, 161, **162**
CT, **163**
with fat necrosis, **163**
chronic, **166**
principles of management, 166
papillary carcinoma, thyroidectomy specimen,
272
papilloma
intraduct, breast, **31**
pedunculated, **44**
paraphimosis, **301**
parathyroid, 274
adenoma, **274**
paronychia, **3**
parotid gland, 77
anatomy, **78**
parotitis, acute, **79**
peau d'orange, **33**
pelvic inflammatory disease, **228**
pelvi-ureteric junction obstruction, **286**
penis, 299–302
carcinoma, **302**
peptic ulceration, 123
perforating veins, calf, **256**
perforator ligation, **256**
peri-ampullary cancer, **167**
perianal abscess, recurrent, **214**
periodontal disease, **73**
peripheral nerve injuries, 331–8
peroneal nerve, common, injury, **338**
phaeochromocytoma, **280**
pharyngeal pouch, **84**
pharynx, 82–3
phimosis, **301**
phlebitis, **13**
pilonodal sinus, **41**
pinch grafting, **258**
pituitary tumour, **317**
pleura, 87–8
pleural effusion, **17**
pneumonia, 86–7
pneumoperitoneum, **127**
pneumothorax, 87, **87**
polyarteritis nodosa, small bowel, **191**
polycystic kidney disease, **284**
polycystic liver disease, **135**
polyp, colorectal
adenomatous, **204**
metaplastic, **204**
polyposis
familial adenomatous, **205**
gastric, **127**

popliteal artery
  aneurysm, **252**
  embolus, **242**
  palpation, **235**
portal hypertension, 139–41
porto-systemic collateral circulation, **140**
postoperative complications, 13–18
pregnancy, ectopic, ruptured, **230**
premalignant conditions, skin, 50
prostate, 298
  carcinoma metastases, **298**
pruritus ani
  differential diagnosis, 210
  excoriation, **211**
pseudocyst, pancreas, **164, 165**
pseudomembranous colitis, **202**
pulmonary atelectasis, **17**
pupil, fixed dilated, **322**
purpura, idiothrombocytopenic, **176**
pyelonephritis, chronic, **287**
pyloric stenosis, 122
  acquired, 126
pyogenic abscesses, **137**
pyrexia, and intra-abdominal abscess, **120**

radial nerve, injury, **333, 334**
radiodermatitis, **35**
ram's horn, 42
ranula, **70**
rash, drug hypersensitivity, **16**
Raynaud's disease, **246**
Recklinghausen's disease, 47
recto-sigmoid junction, carcinoma, obstructing, 207
recto-urethral fistula, **180**
rectum, 209–17
  cancer, stages, 204
  carcinoma, 203, **216**
  prolapse, **215**
  villous adenoma, **216**
renal artery, stenosis, **99**
renal cell carcinoma, **292**
renal colic, **289**
renal cyst, **285**
renal dysplasia, **287**
renal mass, differential diagnosis, 282
renal pelvis, transitional cell carcinoma, **294**
renal trauma, **290**
renal tuberculosis, **288**
retrosternal thyroid, **101**
rhabdomyosarcoma, **52**
rhinorrhea, cerebrospinal fluid, **320**
Richter's hernia, **225**
rodent ulcer, **51**
rule of nines, 9

salivary glands, 77–81
saphena varix, **255**
sarcoma, osteogenic, **76**
scar, keloid, hypertrophic, **12**
sclerotherapy, injection, 255
scrotum
  Fournier's gangrene, **308**
  swelling, differential diagnosis, 304
sebaceous cyst, **21, 39**
Seldinger technique, 239

seminoma, **307**
sialectasis, **79**
sialolithiasis, submandibular gland, **81**
sigmoid volvulus, **186**
skin, 37–58
  benign conditions, 38–42
  premalignant conditions, 50
  tumour, 43–58
    benign, 44–8
    classification, 43
    malignant, 51–2
small bowel, 187–94
  malrotation, **180**
  neoplasm, 192–4
  NSAID-induced diaphragms, **186**
  obstruction, strangulated, **185**
  polyarteritis nodosa, **191**
  volvulus, **180**
somatic pain, 116
spermatic cord, anatomy, **303**
spina bifida occulta, **325**
spinal cord, 325–30
  cervical, whiplash injury, **326**
  lumbar, fracture, **327**
  traumatic compression, **328**
spleen, 173–7
  cyst, **175**
  laceration, **175**
  melanoma, metastatic, **177**
splenic artery, mycotic aneurysm, **177**
splenomegaly, 173
  clinical, **174**
splenunculi, **176**
squamous cell carcinoma, **51**
  anus, **217**
  oesophagus, **108**
squamous cell papilloma, oral mucosa, **67**
Staphylococcus aureus, 2, 3
steal syndrome, subclavian, **244**
stenosis
  carotid artery, **315**
  coronary artery, **98**
  femoral artery, **239, 240**
  iliac artery, **238**
  mitral valve, **96**
  pyloric, 122
    acquired, **126**
  renal artery, **99**
  vein graft, **242**
  vertebral artery, **315**
stitch sinus, **15**
stomach, 121–31
  carcinoma, 128–31
    antral, **130**
  see also gastric
stone formation, kidney, 288
strawberry naevus, **46**
Streptococcus spp., 2, 4, 6
  and periorbital cellulitis, 4
subarachnoid haemorrhage, **313**
subclavian steal syndrome, **244**
subcutaneous tissue, 37–58
subdural haematoma, **324**
sublingual gland, 77
submandibular gland, 77
  sialolithiasis, **81**

subphrenic abscess, 88
subungual melanoma, **56**
superior vena cava, thrombosis, **263**

teratoma, **308**
testis, 303–8
    anatomy, **303**
    maldescent, 304, **304**
    torsion, **305**
    tumours, 307–8
tetanus, 5
thorax, 85–113
thromboangiitis obliterans, **246**
thrombocytopenia, acquired, **176**
thrombosis
    axillary vein, spontaneous, **262, 263**
    deep venous, **16**, 260–4
    superior vena cava, **263**
thrush, oral, **65**
thymoma, **101**
thyroglossal cyst, **23**
thyroid, 266–73
    anatomy, **266**
    neoplasms, 271–3
    retrosternal, **101**
thyroidectomy, 272
    complications, 273
thyroiditis, Hashimoto's, **269**
thyrotoxicosis, **270**
tinker's tartan, 10
toenail, ingrowing, **41**
tongue, 71–3
    aphthous ulcer, **72**
    carcinoma, **73**
    geographic, **72**
    tied, **71**
tonsillitis, acute, **83**
toxic megacolon, **201**
transitional cell carcinoma
    bladder, **296**
    renal pelvis, **294**
transurethral resection of the prostate, 298
trauma
    aortic dissection, **102**
    chest wall, 91
    diaphragmatic hernia, **114**
    hepatic, **136**
    renal, **290**
    spinal cord compression, **328**
Trendelenburg test, **254**
tuberculosis
    disseminated, **8**
    renal, **288**
tumour, *see specific sites and types*
Turner's sign, **162**
TURP, 298

ulcer
    aphthous, tongue, **72**
    duodenal, **123, 124, 125**
    gastric, **125**
    ischaemic, foot, **237**
    malignant, **259**
    Marjolin's, **50**, 259
    oesophagus, **107**
    rodent, **51**

ulceration
    chronic, **50**
    varicose, 257–9
        pinch grafting, **258**
ulcerative colitis, **200**, 200–3
    pathological specimen, **201**
ulcerative tumour, colonoscopy, **206**
ulnar nerve, injury, **336, 337**
umbilical fistula, **187**
umbilical hernia, **218**
ureter, 282–94
    calculus, **289**
    duplication, **285**
urethra, 299–302
    rupture, **300**
    valves, **299**
urinalysis, **118**
urinary retention, **15**
urine, chronic retention, **297**
urology, 281–308

valvular disease, 95–7
varicocele, 306
varicose veins, 253–6
varix
    gastric, **141**
    oesophageal, **141**
vascular disease, 231–64
    multivessel, **98**
vein graft, stenosis, **242**
veins, 253–64
    perforating, calf, **256**
venography, deep venous thrombosis, **261**
venous drainage, leg, **253**
venous insufficiency, chronic, 257–9
venous thrombosis, deep, 260–4
vertebral artery, stenosis, **315**
vertebral body, cervical, metastatic
    destruction, **329**
vesico-ureteric reflux, **286**
villous adenoma, colorectal, **205**
visceral pain, 116
volvulus
    caecum, **186**
    gastric, **127**
    sigmoid, **186**
    small bowel, **180**

warts, anal, **217**
whiplash injury, cervical spine, **326**
Whipple's resection, pancreatic carcinoma, **170**
Wilms' tumour, **291**
wound dehiscence, 14
wound haematoma, **14**
wound infection, **14, 15**
wrist, ganglion, **40**

zygoma, fractured, **60, 61**